The Neural Code of Pitch and Harmony

Harmony is an integral part of our auditory environment. Resonances characterized by harmonic frequency relationships are found throughout the natural world, and harmonic sounds are essential elements of speech, communication and, of course, music.

Providing neurophysiological data and theories that are suitable to explain the neural code of pitch and harmony, the author demonstrates that musical pitch is a temporal phenomenon and that musical harmony is a mathematical necessity based on neuronal mechanisms. Moreover, he offers new evidence for the role of an auditory time constant for speech and music perception as well as for similar neuronal processing mechanisms of auditory and brain waves.

Successfully relating current neurophysiological results to the ancient ideas of Pythagoras, this unique title will appeal to specialists in the fields of neurophysiology, neuroacoustics, linguistics, behavioural biology and musicology, as well as to a broader audience interested in the neural basis of music perception.

Gerald Langner received a diploma in physics from the Technical University of Munich in 1971. He then worked at the Max-Plank Institute in Göttingen and at the TU Darmstadt, where he studied hearing in birds and electroreception in fish. In 1985, during a research stay in Canberra, Australia, he discovered – together with Henning Scheich – the electric sense in platypus. From 1988 to 2008 he was Professor of Neurobiology in Darmstadt, with his research focusing on spatial and temporal aspects of processing in the auditory system.

The Neural Code of Pitch and Harmony

GERALD LANGNER

Technische Universität, Darmstadt, Germany

EDITED BY

CHRISTINA BENSON

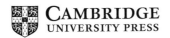

CAMBRIDGE
UNIVERSITY PRESS

University Printing House, Cambridge CB2 8BS, United Kingdom

Cambridge University Press is part of the University of Cambridge.

It furthers the University's mission by disseminating knowledge in the pursuit of education, learning and research at the highest international levels of excellence.

www.cambridge.org
Information on this title: www.cambridge.org/9780521874311

First published 2015

Printed in the United Kingdom by TJ International Ltd. Padstow Cornwall

A catalogue record for this publication is available from the British Library

Library of Congress Cataloguing in Publication data
Langner, Gerald, 1943–
The neural code of pitch and harmony / Gerald Langner, Technische Universität, Darmstadt, Germany ; edited by Christina Benson.
    pages   cm
Includes bibliographical references and subject index.
ISBN 978-0-521-87431-1
1. Bioacoustics.   2. Neurobiology.   3. Sound – Physiological effect.
4. Sound – Psychological aspects.   5. Harmonic analysis (Music)   6. Contentment.
I. Benson, Christina, editor.   II. Title.
QH510.5.L36   2015
612′.014453–dc23
                                                                        2014043973

ISBN 978-0-521-87431-1 Hardback
ISBN 978-0-521-69701-9 Paperback

Contents

Preface

Sound is a vital tool for humans and animals. We communicate with each other through speech, we convey emotion by laughing or crying, but we also purposefully create sounds using our voices or musical instruments just because we perceive them to be appealing or beautiful. The pitch, rhythm and melody of speech and music can communicate emotions like fear, pleasure and anger quite quickly and efficiently. Moreover, as humans we seem to have a powerful urge to fill the world with sounds of our own creation, with the result that these days music surrounds us virtually everywhere. The need to make, listen and dance to music stretches back to the very beginnings of our history: for many thousands of years music has played an essential role in our social interactions, rituals and ceremonies. The sixth-century Roman philosopher and great musical theorist Boethius stated quite simply:

it appears beyond doubt that music is so naturally united with us that we cannot be free from it even if desired.

We all know that some combinations of musical tones sound particularly good when played together or subsequently; we call these 'consonant' or 'harmonious', while others sound harsh or 'dissonant'. If asked what combinations of sounds they find pleasant, or at least interesting, people from different cultural backgrounds may not completely agree. Different forms of music prevail in different regions of the world, and musical instruments and composition have become progressively more sophisticated as civilization advances. Nevertheless, there are certain combinations of tones that seem to have universal appeal. They are preferred everywhere and form the basis of musical systems throughout the world. Clearly, there must be some universal rules that are crucial to our perception of musical harmony.

The question of what these rules are and what might be the role of whole numbers dates back to the time of the ancient Greeks. They believed that the mathematical rules of musical harmony are the very same that govern the entire universe. Besides neurophysiologic data and theories that are suitable to explain auditory processing of pitch and harmony, this book provides new evidence for this ancient philosophical concept. The conclusion is that our sense for musical harmony is an unavoidable consequence of mathematical rules underlying temporal processing in our hearing system. As we progress through this book, theories and models of pitch perception and harmonic perception, both historical and current, will be presented and explained. Finally, in the last chapter I will suggest that neuronal dynamic processes similar to those in the hearing system are involved in other crucial brain functions: motor control, emotion and memory processing.

The book is intended not only for neuroscientists and musicologists, but also for a broader audience interested in the perceptual basis of music. Therefore boxes in various chapters contain additional information that may be helpful, although perhaps unnecessary for the specialist. Moreover, in the times of internet it should be quite easy to obtain additional information for those who want to go into details.

Foreword

Human sensing abilities have been shaped and refined over long evolutionary periods. Hearing has adapted to serve us well in many different tasks and situations, helping us to orient ourselves and to survive in the world. The general properties of peripheral and central mechanisms of hearing are highly conserved across vertebrates due to very similar environmental conditions. Species-specific variations do exist, such as the use of ultrasound for orientation in bats and cetaceans, but they are usually founded on quantitative and not qualitative differences to generally applicable principles of hearing and brain mechanisms. Basic hearing tasks for survival include detecting, localizing and identifying sound sources in cluttered or noisy environments. Another critical role of vertebrate hearing is the control and analysis of communication sounds which, in humans, lead to the highly developed ability of speech production and perception. Speech, like many other sounds involving resonance phenomena, contains harmonic elements, i.e. frequency components that are integer multiples of a common 'fundamental' frequency. These sounds can evoke a perceptual phenomenon, periodicity or virtual pitch that is distinct from other perceptual dimensions of sounds. A most human endeavour, the production and enjoyment of music, is fundamentally based on this perceptual phenomenon. Studies of the brain mechanisms that lead to this perception, its psychophysical manifestation and, eventually, cognitive and emotional benefits have progressed for more than a century, as is outlined in this volume, but still many aspects remain unresolved.

A helpful aspect in resolving this matter may be found in the fact that humans have surrounded themselves with an environment of their own creation. Based on our ability to use tools we have created artificial soundscapes that serve, entertain and move us. Unsurprisingly, many of those sound aspects have been, often inadvertently, chosen to match or most effectively engage our biological sound analysis system. Examples include the choice for frequency transitions in ambulance sirens to catch our attention, or the relationship of voices in polyphonic music. Both of these examples can be traced to specific psychophysically verified and physiologically implemented principles of sound processing. Furthermore, instrumental music is a solely human development that emerged early in our evolution to become human, as indicated by the recovery of Palaeolithic flutes created more than 40 000 years ago. The sound effects emanating from these old – and current, electronic – artefacts of musical sound generation also must reflect and potentially reveal basic properties of our auditory system.

The author of this book has been fascinated by these aspects for a long time and has tried to create a unifying perspective. In the early 1980s, I joined the Coleman Memorial Laboratory at the University of California in San Francisco, which is dedicated to the study of the physiological basis of hearing and deafness. Shortly thereafter, Dr Gerald Langner arrived for his first of many extended visits to explore sound processing in the central auditory system, especially in the auditory midbrain, an obligatory processing station between the inner ear and the auditory cortex. Over the years we embarked on several studies, especially with regard to the processing of amplitude-modulated sounds, a simplified exemplar of a harmonic sound. As a trained physicist, Gerald was keen to approach biological phenomena from a theory-driven perspective. A theory of pitch processing, understood as a construct of hypotheses based on physical, psychophysical and physiological aspects, should be able to provide verifiable predictions of the processing and role of harmonic coding in animals and humans. I recall many discussions of new data points, derived over long days and nights in the laboratory, in which he invoked his credo: 'Never trust data, unless you have a theory.'

In this book the author outlines his conclusions from this lifelong pursuit of potential links between aspects of our neural machinery of pitch processing and their reflection in our self-created sound environment. Drawing on theoretical, computational, physiological, psychophysical and music-historical evidence, he has created a compelling scenario of the properties of some brain mechanisms and their expression in our percepts as well as their reflection in the cultural world we have created around us. He provides a fascinating journey into the history and future of pitch and brain studies and suggests intriguing interactions of fine-scale neural processes in our brain with our cultural history of sound creation.

Christoph E. Schreiner
San Francisco
November 2014

1   Historical aspects of harmony

'Musica est exercitium arithmeticae occultum nescientis se numerare animi.'
    'Music is a hidden arithmetical exercise of the soul, which does not know that it is
dealing with numbers.'

(Gottfried Wilhelm Leibniz, 1646–1716)

1.1   The origin of music

For thousands of years, music has played an essential role in social interactions, rituals and
ceremonies, although its exact origins are shrouded in mystery. From an evolutionary
viewpoint, the desire to produce musical sounds is not unique to man. We are all familiar
with the sound of birds singing. Some non-human primates also sing; monkeys in the
rainforests of Asia and gibbons in the jungles of Thailand produce haunting musical calls:
their duets probably serve to strengthen pair bonding, but singing may also serve to alarm
other group members (Chung and Geissmann, 2000; Geissmann, 2002). If musical sounds
are important in primate communication, they must also have been essential in early human
communication. Perhaps as suggested by Charles Darwin (Darwin, 2004), singing may even
have preceded speech and might have been the primary method of human communication.

One can only speculate as to why our ancestors produced their first musical instruments; it may have been an attempt by early man to imitate natural sounds, such as
the wind blowing through a hollow reed or the singing of a bird. The earliest known
instruments are flutes, made from bone or mammoth ivory, dating back tens of thousands
of years to the Palaeolithic Age. For example, in the Geißenklösterle cave near
Blaubeuren in Germany, archaeologists uncovered the oldest known musical
instrument – a primitive, but carefully constructed, swan-bone flute estimated to be at
least 35 000 years old (Fig 1.1; Hahn and Münzel, 1995; Münzel et al., 2002). Similar
flutes have been found at other locations in Europe, suggesting that music was certainly a
part of Stone Age life (see also Section 5.5).

But more sophisticated forms of music also have ancient roots. We know that lyres with
many strings were in use in ancient Sumeria almost 5000 years ago. The ancient Egyptians
included complex forms of music and dance in their everyday life and religious worship.
Paintings in their tombs and temples show professional musicians and a wide variety of
instruments like lyres, pipes, lutes and drums. Many of these instruments have survived
and may be regarded as predecessors of our modern instruments.

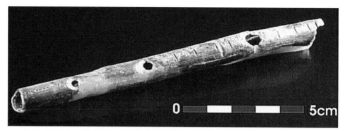

Fig. 1.1   A 35 000-year-old swan-bone flute from the Geißenklösterle cave in Germany
(Conard *et al.*, 2009). Its three holes allow playing harmonic tones, thereby supporting the idea
that our harmonic sense must have biological roots.

1.2   The power of music and harmony

We know that music has been an important part of every culture and civilization
throughout history, but what exactly it represents to us is still a mystery. At some time
we have all experienced the inexplicable and magical power that some forms of music
have over us, but the origin of this power remains elusive. The Austrian author Robert
Musil expresses this enigma in the following way: 'The human mystery of music is
not that it is music, but that with the help of a dried sheep gut it succeeds in bringing us
nearer to God' (Musil, 1982).

It is often said that music 'speaks to our unconscious mind' and, indeed, it may be
more subtle and obscure than all other forms of art. As a rule, music does not provide
us with an identifiable portrayal or, at least, an association to our world, as is often
the case with paintings or sculptures. It is abstract. Yet, when we listen to certain
musical compositions the combinations of melody, harmony and rhythm may evoke
profound, sometimes almost unworldly, emotions within us: 'in its physical effect, in
the way it grabs one by the head and shoulders, it is one of those manifestations of
beauty that border on the 'heavenly' and of which only music and no other art is
capable' (Mann, 1997).

Thomas Mann is expressing the ecstatic feeling of 'musical chills' or 'shivers', a
manifestation of the intense feelings of pleasure which most of us have experienced
when listening to certain pieces of music (Gabrielsson, 2012; see also Section 12.3.2).
Somehow, we are able to transcend reality, to be transported into another world.
Modern imaging techniques have recently been used to map brain activity during
these experiences, and have shown that brain areas associated with reward or euphoria
(intense feelings of happiness) are especially strongly activated (Zatorre, 2003; see
also Section 10.6).

Music also has an exceptionally strong ability to revive old memories. As we listen to
our favourite symphonies, arias or pop songs, the emotions that are aroused may become
united with vivid memories and our mood or even our behaviour may change. It is this
mysterious, almost magical power that has made music a ubiquitous and fundamental
expression of human life. In Chapter 12 I will discuss how this effect of emotional
memory relates to the dynamics and oscillatory activity of our brain.

1.3   Music as a universal language

In a way music, and the harmony within it, could be considered a universal language, a form of communication stretching beyond the barriers of speech. Music has evolved in many different forms throughout the world and, as we all know, even within the same cultural environment musical tastes can be drastically different. Nature, however, has provided us with the perceptual means to understand, and often enjoy, the varied musical traditions of different cultures. Although some aspects of unfamiliar forms of music may sound strange to our ears, all music seems to contain some crucial elements that we can immediately recognize and relate to. A major reason for this is that all humans share not only a similar sense of rhythm and pitch, but also a similar appreciation for musical harmony – that is, for certain harmonic intervals (Stumpf, 1890).

Our perception of these intervals is based on mathematical rules (see also Section 11.8) and, consequently, must be universal. A vivid depiction of this is the final scene of Steven Spielberg's movie *Close Encounters of the Third Kind*. In a clash between civilizations the American army faces an extraterrestrial spaceship at the foot of the Devil's Tower in Wyoming, and the question arises of whether and how these two radically different civilizations might be able to speak to each other.

The seemingly unsolvable communication gap is bypassed by the use of musical signals. The musical language 'Solresol', which bridged the chasm in the movie, was invented in the nineteenth century by Jean-François Sudre. It is based on a seven-note scale where each note acts as an element of language. Indeed, musical scales – the foundation of most musical compositions – are astonishingly similar in all cultures. Although the number of notes may differ, almost all scales are based on two major harmonic intervals: octaves and fifths.

We are able to recognize symmetry, proportion and balance in music, just as we can in visual art. In terms of music, harmony refers to certain relationships between tones of the same (prime) or different pitches. The pitch of a tone may be regarded as a subjective measure of its relative highness or lowness and characterizes its position in the complete range of tones. In our standard Western (diatonic) scale an interval of eight notes (an octave) represents the highest degree of musical harmony or consonance (after the prime). There is an indisputable 'sameness' about two tones an octave apart; they actually sound so similar that they are often confused with primes. For example, men and women singing together 'in unison' are usually singing the same notes an octave apart, although they may not be aware of it (something similar applies to communication signals of certain species of electric fish and mosquitoes; see Section 9.1). Correspondingly, musical systems everywhere, ancient and modern, use the interval of the octave as their indispensable cornerstone.

An interval of five notes (the fifth) is usually considered to be the most consonant interval after the octave and, consequently, is also a universal component of musical systems. The two notes in a fifth do not have the same degree of similarity as those in an octave, but do seem to fuse in a very natural and pleasing way (fusion; Stumpf, 1890).

Harmonically related tones are perceived as consonant when played simultaneously, but they can also be combined in sequences to form melodies. It is clear that we are able to easily recognize such subsequent, harmonically related tones and find them aesthetically pleasing. One may ask what is different or unique about such harmonious sequences of tones and what exactly it is that we are receiving, processing and responding to (see Section 11.7). As far as we know, the first person who addressed these questions was the great mathematician and philosopher Pythagoras, about 2500 years ago.

1.4   Musical harmony and whole numbers

Pythagoras was born on the Greek island of Samos in the middle of the sixth century BC. According to Boethius (AD 480–524), who recorded the story more than 1000 years later (Boethius, 1989), Pythagoras noticed the musical and harmonious sounds that were sometimes produced by a blacksmith and his assistants as they pounded with their hammers on an anvil (Fig. 1.2a). His investigations showed that the sounds of the hammers had a pitch which depended on their weight, the heaviest hammer producing a lower pitch than the lighter ones. However, only some of the hammers produced a pleasant harmonious ringing when struck together. His conclusion was that harmonious sounds rang out only when the weights of the hammers being struck together were in

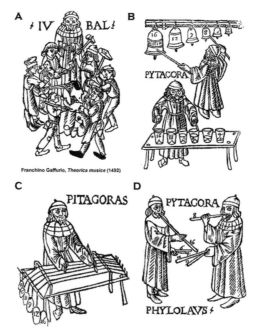

Fig. 1.2   The four drawings show Pythagoras entering the blacksmith's shop **(a)** and exploring the physical basis of pitch and harmony with bells and water-filled tumblers **(b)**, a string instrument **(c)** and with different flutes **(d)** (from *Theorica musice* by F. Gaffurius (1492)).

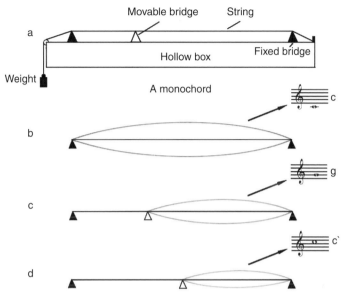

Fig. 1.3   **(a)** The pictured Pythagorean monochord is composed of a single string which is stretched by a weight and supported by three bridges, two fixed and one movable. **(b)** Plucking the whole string produces a certain tone. When the string length is shortened, for example to two-thirds or one-half of its original length, tones a fifth **(c)** or an octave above **(d)** are produced.

simple ratios. Pythagoras had discovered the association between the ratios of small whole numbers and musical consonance.

In order to test his theory, Pythagoras – so the story goes – invented a simple one-stringed instrument known as a monochord (Fig. 1.3). Its movable bridge could be used to change the length of the string and thus the pitch of the tone that was generated. By dividing the string in half (ratio 1:2), the pitch increased by an octave. In addition, Pythagoras found two lesser consonances, the fifth (ratio 2:3) and the fourth (ratio 3:4). Today we know that the pitch of the tone produced is determined by the frequency (periodicity) of vibrations, which changes both with the length and the tension of a string.

Pythagoras realized that musical intervals can be arranged in a hierarchy; those with the ratios of small integers (so-called 'perfect' intervals such as the octave, fifth and fourth) are the most consonant. As the ratio becomes more complex, involving larger numbers, the sound becomes more dissonant. Simpler numerical relationships are thus associated with more pleasant (euphonious) combinations of sounds, revealing a connection between mathematics and aesthetics.

The musical ratios accepted by the Pythagoreans as pleasant (1:2, 2:3 and 3:4) involved only the first four integers. To them, these numbers developed their own mystical meaning; together they form the *tetraktys* (meaning 'fourness'), which was looked upon as a numerical representation of the orderly perfection of the cosmos

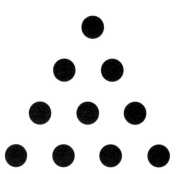

Fig. 1.4   The tetraktys, the symbol of harmony in nature and music, represents the four smallest integers which add up to 10.

(Fig. 1.4). Pythagoreans made an oath on this figure: 'By him who gave to our soul the tetraktys, the source and root of ever-flowing nature.' One can see that all of the three consonance ratios are included in this triangle as adjacent pairs of lines, starting from any of its vertices. Moreover, the sum of the first four integers is 10, which was considered to be of particular significance, a perfect number and a symbol of completeness (wikipedia.org/wiki/Tetraktys).

1.5   Universal harmony

The legend has it that from his pioneering experiments with the vibrating strings of his monochord, Pythagoras had succeeded in establishing a mathematical basis of melodic intonation. In his mind the relationship of whole numbers to musical consonances was seen as a mystery of such great significance that he went on to build an entire philosophical system based on these findings. In his metaphysical concept of 'universal harmony' Pythagoras attempted to explain the whole of creation in terms of numbers and mathematics. He was convinced that the entire universe, including the heavens as well as our minds, is based on a harmony expressed by the same integer relationships as the musical consonances.

Accordingly, the theory of mathematical proportions was a cornerstone of Pythagorean philosophy. It consisted of four pillars – arithmetic, geometry, astronomy and music. Astronomy was interpreted as numbers in motion, geometry as numbers at rest, arithmetic as numbers absolute and music as numbers applied. Of these four disciplines, music was considered to be the only one that directly involves our senses and thus has the potential to influence our behaviour. It is no wonder that the Pythagoreans saw music as a bridge between the transitory world of our physical experience and the eternal laws of nature – a way in which we can subconsciously appreciate the beauty of the mathematical order of the universe.

However, one should not fail to notice that Pythagorean musical theory also had its critics. As time progressed, pure mathematical ideals had become ever more entrenched in the minds of the Pythagoreans and the realities of hearing were increasingly neglected. Practising musicians, in particular, felt that the Pythagoreans were too interested in reducing musical sounds to numerical relationships, and were ignoring what was actually heard; musical harmony had become something to be judged by the intellect, not by the human ear.

Pythagorean number mysticism reached its pinnacle in the metaphysical ideals of Plato (428–347 BC). He stated that human perception must be at fault if musicians did not perform according to mathematical principles. Naturally, such extremely theoretical views provoked antagonism to Pythagorean musical theory. The most vocal critic of Plato's ideas about harmony was the musician Aristoxenus of Tarentum, born in the fourth century BC, and a pupil of Aristotle. His musical philosophy was in stark contrast to Plato's; he felt that a science of music should not be based on physics and mathematics but on the sounds the ear really hears. He dismissed their emphasis on arithmetical relationships as unimportant in terms of music itself: 'harmonic or musical properties attach only to what is heard' (Barker, 2012). In Chapter 11 we will conclude that this may be only an apparent contradiction because in a way the harmonic processing of our hearing system corresponds to mathematical principles.

1.6   Harmony of the Spheres

Pythagoras' idea of a musical–mathematical harmony permeating the universe led to the concept of the 'Harmony of the Spheres', an appealing idea that united music with astronomy. Pythagoras thought of the cosmos as a huge lyre with crystal spheres instead of strings. In this system, the Earth was in the centre and the sun, moon and planets were attached to the crystal spheres. The distances of the planets from Earth were ordered as in a musical scale, with the interval between the Earth and an outer sphere of fixed stars being equal to an octave. The relative speeds of the planets, in accordance with their distances from Earth, were thus in the same proportions as the musical consonances (compare Fig. 1.5). As the planets revolved they each emitted a tone and a wonderfully harmonious sound was produced, the *Musica Mundana*, or 'music of the spheres'. This 'cosmic music', which, as his disciples believed, only Pythagoras could hear, was thought to reveal the sound of the harmony of the creation of the universe (see below). The theme of a harmonically constructed universe was revisited several more times in the ensuing centuries, first by Plato and then most notably in the late sixteenth century by Johannes Kepler (Helmholtz, 1863: p. 375). More recently, Paul Hindemith's opera 'The Harmony of the World' about Kepler focuses on the same idea. In Hindemith's theories of musical harmony, a tonal centre can be identified with the sun and other tones with planets at varying distances from the sun.

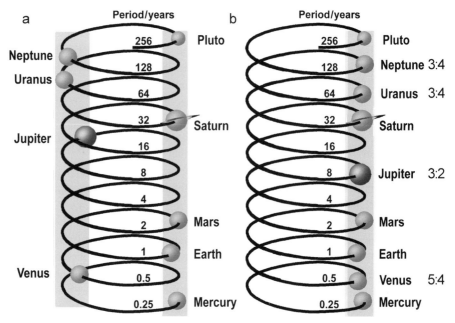

Fig. 1.5 (a) The helix represents the orbital periods of the nine planets of our solar system covering about ten octaves. The exact position of a planet in the helix indicates its period. The periods of neighbouring planets on adjacent arcs would differ by an octave. The periods of Earth and Jupiter differ by three octaves and a fifth with a deviation of only 1%. (b) If one transforms the period of Jupiter by a fifth (2:3), those of Neptune and Uranus by a fourth (3:4) and that of Venus by a major third (4:5), the vertical arrangement reveals that the whole solar system is, to a certain extent, subject to gravitational resonance.

1.7 Harmony in modern astrophysics

Pythagorean number mysticism may seem to us today to be completely metaphysical. It must be emphasized, however, that apparently never before had anyone attempted to describe natural phenomena using mathematics. Pythagoras' emphasis on the importance of whole numbers in the order of nature transformed both science and music theory, and his observations can thus be seen as pioneering the study of natural science as we now know it. As a result of his discoveries, mathematics became inextricably linked with science and philosophy, and science became joined with music. Until the seventeenth century music was considered a branch of science, and scientific experimentation was often directed at solving musical problems.

Nowadays we have become used to scientific reasoning based on experimental observation and it therefore appears remarkable that the Pythagoreans constructed their view of a mathematically governed universe with scarcely any actual evidence. It was not until more than 2000 years later that Sir Isaac Newton formulated his laws of motion and gravitation, and finally showed that the universe could indeed be explained in terms of mathematics.

On the other hand, today we also know that planets do indeed tend to synchronize their travels around the sun. For example, the relations of the periods of Uranus, Neptune and Pluto are quite close to 1:2:3 (84, 164, 248 years). Also, the moons of Jupiter have orbital periods in nearly octave relationships, namely 1, 2, 4 and about 8 times 1.8 days (Murray and Dermott, 1999).

It has been known for centuries that the planetary orbits of our solar system are regularly spaced – this was described by an empirical rule, the 'Titius–Bode law'. Astrophysicists believe that this empirical law is most likely based on resonance (the preference for a certain oscillation frequency), or near resonance, of the periodic movements of the planets around the sun (Dermott, 1973; Torbett *et al.*, 1982).

The extent to which our solar system is resonating may be visualized by means of a helix with ten turns: the helix in Fig. 1.5a covers periods from 0.24 to 256 years, where each turn represents a certain octave. Symbols for planets are shown at locations corresponding to their periods. As the figure shows, planets whose periods differ by about one or more octaves ($1:2^n$, n = 1, 2, 3 ...) line up roughly along vertical chains. There are two chains located on opposite sides of the helix; the underlying grey bars on opposite sides are separated by about a fifth in addition to the vertical octave. However, the periods of all planets (with the exception of Neptune and Pluto) differ by larger intervals including additional octaves, fifths, fourths and thirds. More precisely, if one ignores octaves a Jupiter is separated from the Earth-group (Mercury, Earth, Mars, Saturn, Pluto) by a fifth (3:2), Neptune and Uranus by a fourth (4:3) and Venus by a major third (5:4). If one transforms the periods of Jupiter, Neptune, Uranus and Venus, they differ by about one or several octaves and, accordingly, all symbols of planets line up roughly vertically (Fig. 1.5b). Obviously, to a first approximation, the whole solar system from Mercury to Pluto is subject to gravitational resonances and, as a consequence, to some extent obeys simple harmonic rules.

Furthermore, the 2006 Nobel Prize for Physics was awarded to John Mather and George Smoot for their measurements of the 'cosmic microwave background radiation'. Extremely precise measurements of the temperature (to one part in 10^5) of this cosmic radiation have shown that 'the early universe resounded with harmonious acoustic oscillations' (Hu and White, 2004). The harmonic sound waves were connected with cosmic radiation, which could escape only 400 000 years after the Big Bang, when neutral atoms were built. Since they could not absorb the electromagnetic waves the harmonic echo of the Big Bang can still be measured today in the sky (Fig. 1.6).

Many scientific developments join that of the cosmic symphony. For instance, the theory of strings postulates that the smallest ultimate particles of our world resemble vibrating strings. Obviously, the idea of cosmic harmony, including the role of resonance and ratios of small integers, is still alive. In this respect, Pythagoras was obviously right. But what about the complementary part of his philosophy: is there indeed a particular role for resonance and small integers in our mind? If we could understand the neuronal basis of pitch perception, would it clarify the role of numbers and ratios for the perception of harmony? Could the association between consonance and simple ratios

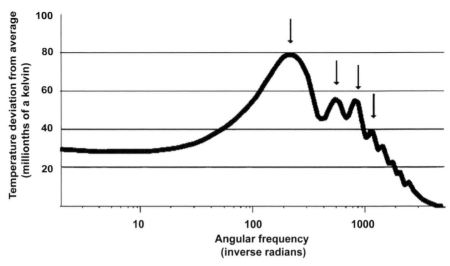

Fig. 1.6   Tiny temperature differences of cosmic microwave radiation across the sky reveal the harmonic acoustic vibrations of the universe 'shortly' after the Big Bang. The first peak in the power spectrum is caused by the fundamental frequency of the 'echo' of the early universe; the subsequent peaks show the effects of the overtones (see arrows; modified from Hu and White, 2004).

be explained by the way nerve cells in our auditory system process pitch information and by the way they react to harmonic sounds? And, moreover, is there also a possible role of resonance and harmony in non-auditory systems of the brain?

These are the final questions that are addressed in Chapters 11 and 12 of this book. But first, some historic facts and basic knowledge about sound is presented in Chapter 2, while Chapters 3 and 4 are devoted to key historical developments and discoveries which have formed the foundation of modern theories of pitch perception. Chapter 5 will offer some new evidence for an auditory time constant and its role in animal communication, speech and music. Moreover, after an introduction to the neurobiology of our hearing system (Chapter 6) the subsequent chapters provide essential research results and theories concerning the neuronal processing mechanisms (Chapters 7–9) and the spatial representation (Chapter 10) of pitch.

2 Sound and periodicity

'A musical sound is produced by pulses or waves which follow each other at regular intervals with sufficient rapidity of succession.'

(John Tyndall, 'Sound', Lecture II, Longmann & Co., 1893)

2.1 Sound is movement

The Ancient Greeks had only a limited understanding of the physical nature of sound, but they did realize that sound is produced by the movement of an object or of parts of an object. They also knew that the pitch of the sound is related to certain physical attributes of the sound-emitting object, such as its weight or its length. Archytas of Tarentum, in the fourth century BC, may have been the first to make the connection between the vibration frequency of an object and the pitch of the resulting sound. Aristotle (384–322 BC) noticed the phenomenon of resonance in strings, and even observed that the tone of a vibrating string contains the octave of its fundamental pitch. Yet for thousands of years the mechanisms behind the creation of harmonic sounds, i.e. the periodic oscillations of strings or other vibrating structures, remained a mystery.

In addition, very little was known of the means by which sound propagates, how it is transmitted through the air to reach our ears. Aristotle compared echoes with balls bouncing back from a wall and correctly concluded that sound must travel by means of waves. Almost 2000 years later, Leonardo da Vinci (1452–1519) also concluded that sound propagates just like waves in water – he compared acoustical echoes to the reflection of waves on the banks of a pond.

In the seventeenth century, the British scientist Robert Boyle (1626–1691) convincingly demonstrated for the first time that sound needs a medium, such as air, to propagate. From his experiments it became clear that the vibration of a membrane, a tube or a string elicits corresponding oscillations of adjacent molecules in the air. The oscillatory movement of the air molecules adds to their Brownian (heat) motion and gives rise to changes in air density and pressure which in turn cause the movement of further molecules. The molecules do not actually travel, but oscillate about their equilibrium position, and the resulting vibration spreads through the air (or another medium) as waves of pressure fluctuations (Fig. 2.1). The velocity of sound is proportional to the sound frequency (f) and wavelength (λ): $c = \lambda \cdot f$. Since the molecules move forth and back and in the same direction as the wave propagates, sound waves are called

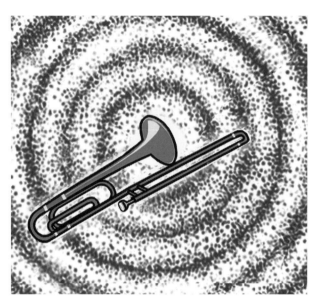

Fig. 2.1   A periodic sound wave, as produced by a trombone, is transmitted through the air by periodic interactions of air pressure, air density and movement of air molecules.

'longitudinal waves'. Light waves, in contrast, are transverse waves that are carried by the oscillations of electromagnetic fields in a direction orthogonal to that of their propagation.

After their transmission through the air, the mechanical vibrations are picked up by our eardrum and ear bones, and finally reach the nerve cells in our inner ear. There, so-called 'hair cells' transfer them into corresponding electrochemical signals and send them as a spatio-temporal excitation pattern to the neurons of our central auditory system (see Section 6.2). As a result we can even hear, for example, the variations in a tone caused by minute movements of a finger on a violin string, or the subtle emotional alterations of the pitch and periodicity of somebody's vocal cords.

2.2   The periodicity of sound

2.2.1   Nature of periodic sounds

Acoustic signals are present in endless diversity. In contrast to signals of other sensory domains, they may be considered as primarily temporal signals. Visual signals, in comparison, are often completely stationary; temporal variations, which are actually indispensable to avoid sensory adaptation, have to be added by the slow and fast movements of our eyes. The main reason for visual stationarity is that our main light sources, the sun and – nowadays – electric lights, are usually of reliable constancy. We may close our eyes and when we open them again, nothing may have changed. If, on the other hand, we had to rely exclusively on fires and flickering candle lights, the temporal domain would certainly be much more important for our vision.

Acoustic signals always indicate moving objects, which quite often means vibrating objects. Therefore the principal dimension of our hearing is time and temporal variations of our environment are the main message of acoustic signals.

One can basically distinguish two categories of sounds: periodic and non-periodic. Typical examples of non-periodic sounds are those of the wind in the trees, of falling water drops in rain or waterfalls and the rumbling of tumbling stones. Usually such sounds are characterized by irregular repetitions of more or less similar sound events, which sum up to variable fluctuations of sound pressure. They constitute what we generally simply call 'noise'. There are also some special types of non-periodic signals in which at least some aspects are regular; the best-known example of this is perhaps 'white noise', which on average contains all audible frequencies at the same amplitude.

For humans and other creatures that use sound for communication, periodic sounds play a special role. When we perceive such regularly timed acoustic signals we assume that something or someone is operating under very well-defined physical conditions. Therefore, in most cases when we hear a regular clicking, beating or drumming sound we tend to assume it arises from a living sound source. Sometimes this assumption may be misleading, as a famous example from radio-astronomy shows. In 1967 the discovery of a periodic extraterrestic radio signal was received with great enthusiasm by some scientists because its regularity seemed to indicate intelligent life on another planet. But, rather disappointingly, it turned out to 'simply' be the discovery of the first sample of some very strange stellar objects called 'pulsars'.

Periodic signals are abundant in nature and are utilized in many different types of animal communication. Typical examples are the rhythmic tapping of woodpeckers, the regular rattling sound produced by storks with their beaks and the more refined technique used by crickets to 'sing' – by rubbing their wings and legs against each other. From a human perspective, the most important periodic signals arise from the vibrations of vocal cords of humans or animals, or are generated by musical instruments.

2.2.2 Perception of periodic sounds

Clearly, there must be corresponding mechanisms in the hearing systems of animals and humans that are capable of analysing this kind of information. Indeed, neuronal circuits in the brains of various animals, from crickets (Schildberger, 1984) to monkeys (Fishman *et al.*, 2001), have been found that are adjusted to detect periodic signals and to perform a neuronal periodicity analysis.

We do not know, and it is a really difficult philosophical question, what animals actually perceive when their neurons are activated, for example by periodic signals. But we do know what we perceive when we hear such sounds at different repetition rates. Acoustic events in a slow sequence will stimulate our hearing system one after another. Apart from certain adaptation effects, the first event will sound like the last one and – as we know from neurophysiological experiments – the activated neurons will respond correspondingly. For low repetition rates, this holds even for nerve cells in our auditory cortex, the highest processing centre of our hearing system (Schreiner and Langner, 1988). They may respond in the same way to each individual acoustic event and, as a result, we perceive such a sequence as more or less identical and separated events. To a certain extent this may hold up to about 100 events per second, although the percept will then appear increasingly as somewhat 'rough' or 'raspy'. Between about 10 and 100 events per second we can no longer count the number of them, but we still have the feeling that they are separable, at least in principle. Above this range the sound is perceived as more and more contiguous and 'smooth'.

As discussed above, there are two possibilities: either the repetition of a sound event is regular or it is irregular. An irregular sequence we perceive as more or less rough or just noisy, but if the sound is regular or periodic, we are somehow able to recognize the periodicity of these repetitions. Even when the repetition rate is so fast that we can no longer follow the sound events one by one, we can distinguish the repetition period of one sound from that of another sound and we can put a 'label' on it. So, in spite of the fact that we are not able to count the number of events impinging on our ear, once there are more than about 16 events per second, our hearing system is somehow able to determine its repetition rate. We call this perceptual attribute of a periodic sound its 'pitch'.

Already Robert Hooke (1635–1703), one of the most versatile natural philosophers of his time, demonstrated that musical sounds may result from fast periodic tapping noises. According to Birch's *History of the Royal Society* (1757) Hooke used a rapidly rotating brass wheel with regularly spaced teeth. By touching the teeth with a paper card he created sounds with a pitch that varied with the speed of the wheel (Fig. 2.2). This allowed him to determine, for example, the frequency of the wing beats of a mosquito. He also varied the sizes of the teeth in regular intervals to produce sounds of vocal character.

Hooke's acoustic experiments convincingly demonstrated that regular sequences of sound pulses are all that is necessary to produce a musical sound with a well-defined pitch. Two hundred years later, in the nineteenth century, the English physicist John Tyndall (1893) explained it thus:

The only condition necessary to the production of a musical sound is that the pulses should succeed each other in the same interval of time. No matter what its origin may be, if this condition is fulfilled the sound becomes musical. If a watch, for example, could be caused to tick with sufficient rapidity – say one hundred times a second – the ticks would lose their individuality and blend to a musical tone. And if the strokes of a pigeon's wings could be accomplished at the same rate, the progress of the bird through the air would be accompanied by music.

2.3   Fourier analysis

Even if periodic signals have the same period and therefore also the same pitch, they may nevertheless sound quite different. Acousticians sum up everything besides pitch,

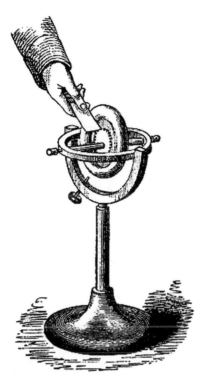

Fig. 2.2   Robert Hooke (1635–1703) realized that a paper card pressed on a rotating brass wheel may be used to produce periodic sound signals (Tyndall, 1893).

loudness and spatial direction that may distinguish two sounds as 'timbre'. The American National Standards Institute defines timbre as: 'that attribute of auditory sensation in terms of which a listener can judge that two sounds similarly presented and having the same loudness and pitch are dissimilar'.

The first 10–50 milliseconds of sounds, the onsets, are especially important for their timbre (Rossing, 1989). Without these onsets a trumpet would sound like a violin and if the tones of a piano are temporally reversed they seem to originate from an organ instead of a piano. But even if one ignores onset effects, tones with the same pitch may still sound entirely dissimilar. At first glance the reason seems quite obvious: in spite of the same pitch, the waveforms of tones, played for example by different musical instruments, may be quite dissimilar. So if the periods of the waveforms shown in Figs. 2.3–2.8 are the same, their pitch will be equal, but not their timbre. However, the physicist and physiologist Herman von Helmholtz (1821–1894) realized that the temporal shape of a signal is not really the crucial factor for the timbre of a sound; he describes this in his famous book *On the Sensations of Tone* (Helmholtz, 1863, 1954; see Chapter 3). In general, different signals have also different frequency compositions (Figs. 2.5–2.8) and this is what really determines their timbre. In contrast, a change of a waveform without a

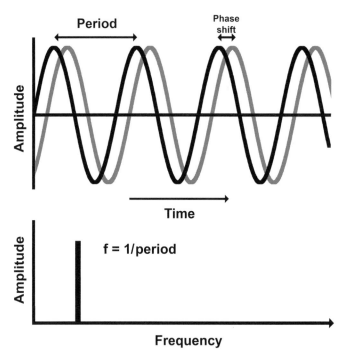

Fig. 2.3   A sine wave is determined by its maximal amplitude, frequency (number of cycles/second) or, alternatively, its period (duration of a cycle), and by its phase. As an example, the two presented signals are shifted in phase.

change of the corresponding frequency compositions (due to phase changes; see below) does not or only scarcely change the timbre.

In order to understand how frequency compositions are related to the waveform of sounds, we have to make use of a certain mathematical tool known as 'Fourier analysis'. Jean Baptiste Joseph Fourier (1768–1830), a French physicist and mathematician, invented this mathematical technique during his investigations of heat conduction (Fourier, 1822). He discovered that he could replace the intricate functions he needed to describe the propagation of heat by simple trigonometric functions. His still indispensable procedure allows one to simplify the analysis of periodic waves (see Box 2.1). They can be replaced by a sum of sine waves of different frequencies, phases and amplitudes, and thus the remarkably simple properties of sine waves can be used to describe and compute how more complex waves propagate in space. The physicist Georg Simon Ohm (1789–1854) – after whom the unit of electrical resistance is named – recognized that Fourier analysis may also be quite appropriate to describe essential aspects of auditory processing, especially the analysis of frequency in the cochlea, the first processing centre of the hearing system.

Fig. 2.3 shows the fundamental properties of a sine wave. This function describes, for example, the movement of a pendulum or, in more general terms, the oscillation of a 'harmonic oscillator'. The parameters of a sine wave are the amplitude – that in

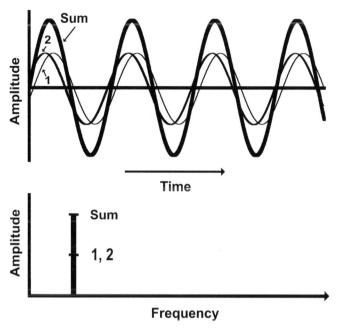

Fig. 2.4   If one adds two sine waves with the same frequencies, the result is another sine wave with the same frequency. The maximal amplitude of the sum depends on the maximal amplitudes and also on the relative phase of the two original sine waves. It is zero when the phases differ by 180 degrees (half a cycle).

sound waves represents sound pressure – or energy and the frequency which counts the number of cycles per second. The complementary parameter of frequency (f) is the period (= 1/f) which indicates the duration of a cycle. As depicted in Fig. 2.3, sine waves may also have different phases; in superpositions this results in different waveforms. But as was shown by Hermann von Helmholtz, our hearing is barely affected by phase changes.

The superposition of two or more sine waves with the same frequency results in another sine wave that has a different amplitude and, in general, also a different phase than the original waves (Fig. 2.4), but its frequency will be the same. If two waves are superimposed that have different frequencies (Fig. 2.5), then sometimes a wave peak will meet another wave peak or a trough, with the result that the amplitude is some-times large and sometimes small or even zero. The greater the difference between the two frequencies, the more quickly this proceeds. Actually, the frequency of the resulting beat is equal to the difference of the two original frequencies. If the two sine waves are two adjacent frequency components of a harmonic sound, the super-position will beat with a frequency that corresponds to the fundamental frequency of the sound, even if this frequency is spectrally 'missing'.

Creating complex signals from sine waves is called Fourier synthesis. Fourier showed that this synthesis is one-to-one, that is, one can produce an arbitary waveform

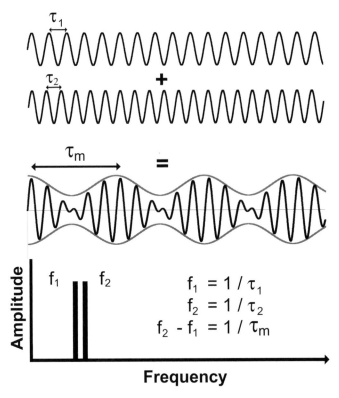

Fig. 2.5   The summation of two sine waves with frequencies f_1 and f_2 gives rise to a waveform, which beats
with the period $\tau_m = 1 / (f_2 - f_1)$. If the frequency difference $f_2 - f_1$ is smaller than 100 Hz the
resulting signal sounds rough, with more or less clear fluctuations of loudness if below 30 Hz and a
pitch, if above 30 Hz (Tartini pitch, see Section 3.5).

in only one way from a sum of different sine waves. Using Fourier analysis, one can
then also resolve the signal into only these same components. A complex periodic
signal (see Fig. 2.7) can be resolved into a number of sine waves with frequencies that
are all integer multiples of the fundamental frequency (the reverse of the signal
period).

By modulating the amplitude of a sine wave (carrier frequency f_c) with another
(modulation frequency f_m) one obtains a sinusoidal amplitude modulation
(AM signal). Another way to generate the same signal is to sum up three sine waves
(f_c, $f_c + f_m$, $f_c - f_m$). If, as shown in Fig. 2.6, the amplitude ratio of the sidebands and the
carrier frequency equals 0.5, the modulation depth of the AM (see arrow) is 100%. The
figure depicts the case where the carrier frequency is an integer multiple of the modulation frequency. Therefore, the difference between the carrier frequency and the sidebands corresponds to the fundamental frequency of the (harmonic) sound. If this
difference is larger than 30 Hz, the AM signal has a (periodicity) pitch that equals that
of its fundamental frequency.

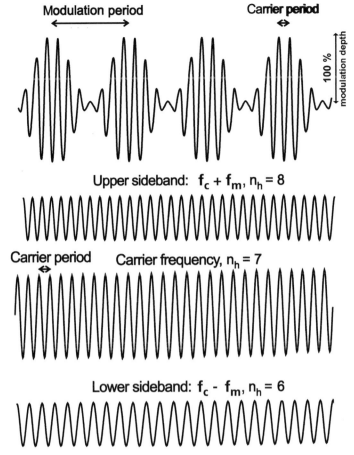

Fig. 2.6 A sinusoidal amplitude modulation (AM signal) results if the amplitude of a sine wave (carrier frequency f_c) is modulated with a modulation frequency (f_m). The same signal may be obtained by just adding three sine waves (f_c, $f_c + f_m$, $f_c - f_m$).

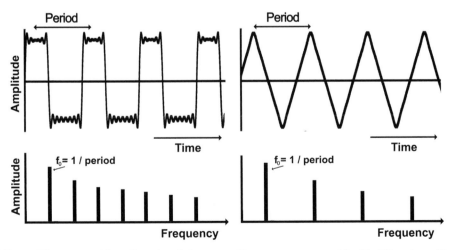

Fig. 2.7 The superposition of a series of sine waves (frequency components) with different amplitudes and phases produces different waveforms. The depicted two signals (top) have the same envelope period and therefore also the same pitch, although they have quite different spectra (bottom). Their period is equal to that of their fundamental frequency. Changing the phases of frequency components changes the shape but not the period of a waveform.

2.4   Sounds of speech

2.4.1   Production of speech

Human speech sounds have broadband spectra in which periodic components, that is, vowels and voiced consonants, alternate with noise or unvoiced consonants (Hartmann, 1997). Voiced speech signals arise through periodic vibrations of the vocal cords and (normally) have a clear pitch (Fig. 2.8). Women have smaller vocal cords and therefore their pitches are on average an octave higher than those of men (about 200 Hz versus about 100 Hz). Since the pitch of vowels, but not their identity, is defined solely through the vibration of the vocal cords, we can speak or sing a certain vowel at different pitches, without changing its identity.

In the larynx the amplitude of overtones of a voiced signal decreases strongly with frequency. Through the adjustable resonance space of the vocal tract some overtones are strengthened more than others. These frequency regions of maximal strengthening are called formants (Figs. 2.8, 2.9). We perceive different combinations of formants as different vowels. While the lower two formants are sufficient to define the vowel, the higher formants are characteristic features of a speaker. The shape of the vocal tract, most importantly the opening of the mouth, the lips and the position of the tongue are important factors that determine the quality or timbre (formants) of a voice. For example, for the same vowels female formants are generally slightly higher than those of men.

Trained opera singers can dominate a whole orchestra by their 'singer's formant' that is absent or only weak in speech or in the spectra of untrained singers. It is this increase in energy at 2500–3000 Hz which allows singers to be heard and understood over an orchestra, which peak at much lower frequencies of around 500 Hz.

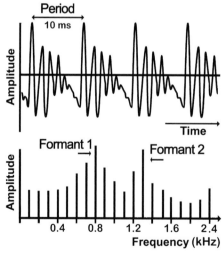

Fig. 2.8   The figure shows the periodic waveform and the spectrum of the vowel *a*, uttered by a male speaker. Although the waveform of a voiced speech signal looks quite complex due to the resonance of the mouth cavities, its period is still defined by the vibration of the vocal cords. The frequencies of the resonance peaks (formants) allow one to distinguish between different vowels.

BOX 2.1 Fourier analysis

If for a certain time interval τ and every time point t a signal $s(t)$ fulfils the condition

$$s(t) = s(t + \tau)$$

it is called periodic with the fundamental period τ. For harmonic perception by the hearing system (Chapter 11) it is important that this implies that periodic signals also repeat themselves with multiples of this fundamental period

$$s(t) = s(t + n\tau), \, n = 1, 2, 3 \ldots .$$

Essential for Fourier analysis are the so-called sine and cosine or circular functions. They may be used, for example, to express the vertical and horizontal coordinates of an object which rotates with a constant speed around a circle. Its angle α (see Fig. 2.1.1) changes with time ($\alpha = \omega \bullet t$). If the object needs the time τ to run around the circle and to increase the angle α by 2π (in radian measure or 360° in degrees), then it holds that

$$2\pi = \omega\tau = 2f\pi\tau, \text{ with } \tau = 1/f.$$

Each period corresponds to $1/f$ seconds; therefore the frequency f is the number of cycles per second.

Now, Fourier's idea was that under certain conditions (that in practice are always fulfilled) each periodic signal may be represented by a sum of sine and cosine functions

$$s(t) = a_0/2 + \sum_{n}^{\infty} (a_n\cos(n\omega t) + b_n \sin(n\omega t))$$

with the coefficients

$$a_0 = \frac{1}{\tau} \int_{-\tau/2}^{+\tau/2} s(t)\, dt, \; a_n = \frac{1}{\tau} \int_{-\tau/2}^{+\tau/2} s(t)\cos(n\omega t)\, dt, \text{ and } b_n$$

$$= \frac{1}{\tau} \int_{-\tau/2}^{+\tau/2} s(t)\sin(n\omega t)\, dt \text{ and } n = 0, 1, 2, 3\ldots .$$

Besides the (possible) constant offset $a_0/2$, every periodic signal can be resolved into a fundamental with a frequency $f = \omega/2\pi$ and additional harmonics with frequencies of 2f, 3f, 4f, etc. Sine and cosine functions of the same frequency add to another circular function with the same frequency, but a different phase (compare Figs. 2.3, 2.4). The amplitudes and phases of these circular functions (harmonics) depend on the signal waveform. The phases may be often largely ignored – as by our hearing system – and (periodic) signals then appropriately represented just in the frequency domain, as amplitudes over frequencies or as a spectrum (see Fig. 2.8). It is important that the Fourier analysis may be applied even to (time limited) non-periodic signals by repeating them periodically.

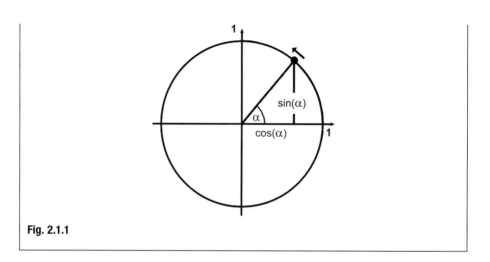

Fig. 2.1.1

2.4.2   Perception of speech

Fig. 2.9 shows a sonagram of the vowels [o:] and [e:], uttered by a male speaker, first analysed with a narrowband (left side; bandwidth 100 Hz) and then by a broadband filter (right side; bandwidth 300 Hz). The narrowband analysis (left) shows that a vowel is composed of a fundamental frequency and harmonics (integer multiples of the fundamental). The broadband analysis (right) reveals the vowel formants (F_1 and F_2) and the period of the fundamental frequency. As a result of the beating of adjacent harmonics the periodicity of the fundamental is indicated over the whole spectral range by vertical stripes (right side).

Vowels can be represented in a 'vowel diagram' in which the second formant (F_2) is plotted over the first one (F_1). Typically, the vowels of a language are arranged in such a diagram in an area known as a 'vowel triangle' with the vowels /i/, /u/ and /a/ at its corners (Kuhl *et al.*, 1997). The vowel formants of different languages are more or less diverse. However, if one plots a sufficient number of them, a triangle can be constructed which encloses nearly all data points (Fig. 2.10). Surprisingly, the corners of this triangle correspond to formant periods that are integer multiples (1, 2, 3 for F_2; 4, 8, 10 for F_1) of a time constant of 0.4 ms. More evidence for the impact of such a time constant will be presented in Chapters 5, 8 and 9, together with a theoretical interpretation.

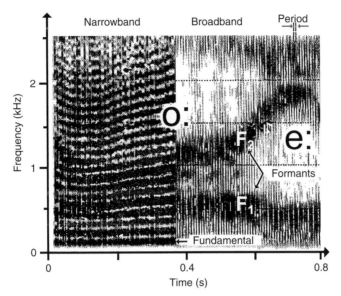

Fig. 2.9 The narrowband spectro-temporal analysis (sonagram) of a speech signal shows its harmonics (dark bands; left side); the corresponding broadband analysis reveals its formats (right side).

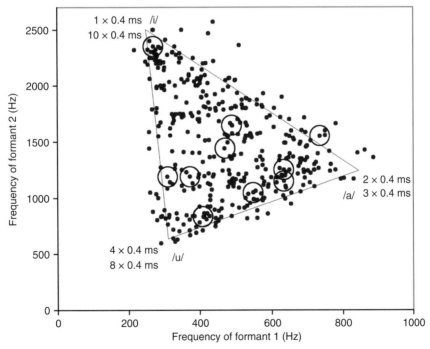

Fig. 2.10 The points in this graph indicate the first two formants of 413 vowels from a total of 25 languages (collected from different internet pages). They are arranged in an area known as the 'vowel triangle'. Most of the points are located within (or close to) a triangle with corners characterized by signal periods that are integer multiples of 0.4 ms (see also Chapter 5). Note the open circles show the location of English vowels.

3 The discovery of the missing fundamental

'Wodurch kann über die Frage, was zu einem Tone gehöre, entschieden werden, als eben durch das Ohr?'
'How else can the question of what belongs to a tone be decided, than by the ear?'
(August Seebeck, Über die Definition des Tones, 1844)

3.1   The sound of sirens

At the beginning of the nineteenth century, the field of experimental acoustics was floundering. One of the main problems at this time was a purely technical one – there was no easy method to vary the frequency of tones in a precise and reproducible way. Experimental research relied on the use of tuning forks or oscillating strings, or on simple musical instruments such as flutes and, in practice, these methods were imprecise and somewhat difficult to handle. Therefore no great progress could be made in understanding the essence and perception of tones.

A turning point for acoustical research came with the invention of the siren as a scientific instrument. Originally introduced by Charles Caignard de la Tour (1819), the siren made it possible to generate tones of a precise and quantifiable frequency. It was this new-found accuracy and reproducibility in tone production which opened the door for acoustics to become both an independent and an exact science.

Several prominent researchers invented their own versions of the siren for acoustical experimentation – one of them, a young German physicist named August Seebeck (Fig. 3.1), constructed a siren which incorporated a number of improvements over Caignard's original design (Fig. 3.2 shows a simple version). It allowed the creation of continuous, clear, steady tones over a large range of pitches. The tones were easily reproducible and could also be quantitatively defined by means of a mechanical counter. Moreover, since the tones were related to the geometric arrangement of the holes on a rotating disc, octaves and other harmonic intervals could be simultaneously generated with high precision. Seebeck's polyphonic siren was subsequently used by several other German scientists, most notably Hermann von Helmholtz, who presented it as the first figure in his treatise on hearing (Helmholtz, 1863).

In 1841 Seebeck used his siren to perform a series of fundamental experiments, the conclusions of which revolutionized our understanding of what constitutes a tone. Seebeck found that tones with a frequency ratio of two would always generate sounds

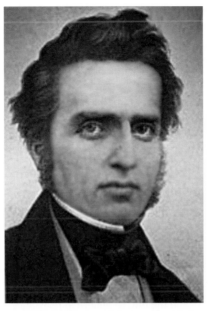

Fig. 3.1   August Seebeck (1805–1849), a director of the Dresden University of Technology, performed a series of pivotal experiments that revolutionized our understanding of what constitutes a tone (from http://tu-dresden.de).

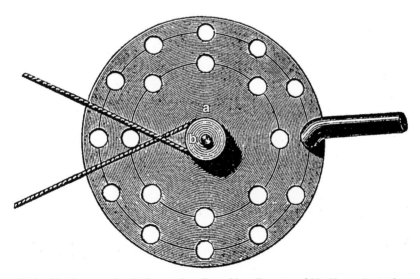

Fig. 3.2   Seebeck's siren consisted of a rotating disc with a diameter of 30–40 cm. A steady stream of air entered through a narrow tube and, as the disc rotated, was blown successively through small holes located at regular distances around its circumference (from Helmholtz, 1863: p. 21).

in an octave relationship; this was independent of the rotation speed of the disc and therefore independent of the absolute value of the generated pitches.

By listening to the siren rather than to oscillating strings, it became obvious, at least to Seebeck, that the pitch of a certain sound was the result of the periodicity of the sound pulses that were generated as the stream of air passed through the individual holes. It was clear that the temporal interval, or period, by which a wave repeats itself had to be the crucial parameter in determining the pitch of the generated sound. Moreover, the sounds produced by his siren convinced Seebeck that the precise shape of the sound pulses must be irrelevant for the pitch and essential only for the timbre of a sound.

3.2   The pitch quarrel

Seebeck's far-reaching conclusions quickly encountered strong opposition; Georg Simon Ohm (see Section 2.3 and Fig. 3.3) was the first to openly reject Seebeck's simple explanations of pitch perception. To most of us Ohm's name is familiar from his law of electrical conduction and the unit of electrical resistance, but he is also renowned for his acoustical research. Since his ideas about the perception of tones were, unfortunately, strongly at odds with those of Seebeck, an increasingly bitter dispute arose between the

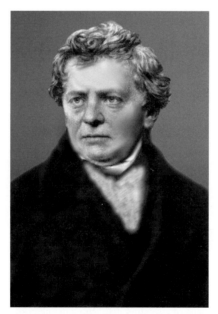

Fig. 3.3   Georg Simon Ohm (1789–1854) was professor of physics at the Polytechnical School of Nuremberg. His law of electric conduction stated the correspondence of voltage and current, his acoustic law that of pure tones and pitches.

two scientists (Turner, 1977). Ultimately, this disagreement led to Ohm's permanent withdrawal from the field of experimental acoustics but, before he pulled out, Ohm, based on the ideas of David Bernoulli (1700–1782), proposed a law known as *Ohm's acoustic law*. It postulated the equivalence of pure tones and pitches and has exerted a strong hold on acoustical science until the present time (see below).

What exactly were the differences between the viewpoints of Ohm and Seebeck? Both agreed that vibrating strings, pipes or other sound sources produce a fundamental frequency as well as additional vibrations of sinusoidal shape – the overtones or harmonics. But Ohm thought that these additional components existed independently from the fundamental; when strong enough they could be heard separately and they in no way interfered with the perception of the fundamental itself. He believed that the pitch, the perceptual label by which a tone received its identity, was defined by each sinusoidal acoustic wave separately, just as waves in the water run across each other but may still be recognized as separate waves. The idea that our hearing system responds to a complex sound by separating out the individual sinusoidal components is the basis of Ohm's acoustic law, which makes use of the principles of Fourier analysis (see Box 2.1).

In 1843, two years after Seebeck had reported his siren experiments, Ohm published a paper in which he appears to be rather shocked that Seebeck had challenged the principle that a certain pitch is always related to a sinusoidal waveform. Ohm was convinced that Seebeck was mistaken when he claimed that the pitch of a sound is evoked merely through the regular repetition of *any* kind of sound pulse, while its precise shape is irrelevant. For Ohm it was out of the question that a wave with a non-sinusoidal shape, produced by a siren, could be wholly responsible for the generation of a clear tone with a definite pitch.

Ohm also refused to believe that Seebeck could hear the same pitch even when the fundamental frequency of the siren was weak, and concluded that Seebeck must be the victim of a '*Gehörstäuschung*' (an auditory illusion). He was convinced that only the fundamental can be responsible for the pitch of the signal. To prove this conjecture, he presented a detailed paper containing a computation of a wave that could be generated by a siren. Much to his satisfaction, the computational result showed that the fundamental component of such a wave has an infinite amplitude. Although Ohm realized that this was physically impossible, he decided that his strange result was nevertheless sufficient to conclude that the fundamental must be the dominant component in the sound of a siren.

Seebeck carefully studied Ohm's paper and, sure enough, discovered a fatal flaw. The 'infinite amplitude of the fundamental frequency' was nothing less than a simple computational error. In absolute contrast to Ohm's bold conclusion, Seebeck's computation showed that the overtones should actually be even more intense than the fundamental. Seebeck, obviously aware how very embarrassing his discovery was for his prestigious opponent, wrote a paper laden with compliments and containing some evidence in support of Ohm's interpretation. He then, however, pointed out the failure of Ohm's theory and drew attention to his critical mathematical error. Ohm was forced to admit his error, but still insisted that Seebeck must have been the victim of an auditory illusion and that our ear must perceive the fundamental of a siren's tone as stronger than it really is and its overtones as weaker than they really are. With this mysterious statement, the embarrassed Ohm completely withdrew from the science of sounds, leaving Seebeck, for a time at least, the acknowledged winner of this acrimonious dispute.

Quite in contrast to Ohm, Seebeck concluded that it is the periodic repetition of sound pressure created by the summed action of the harmonics that is dominant for the pitch of the siren's tone. Furthermore, the fundamental may even be completely missing from the spectrum without changing the pitch of the signal: Seebeck had discovered what was later known as the '*missing fundamental*' phenomenon (Schouten, 1970; see below).

Although Seebeck was essentially right, it was Ohm's hypothesis which ultimately took a firm hold over the field of acoustical research. For well over a century it became the prominent explanation of how we perceive pitch. Even nowadays, many scientists and musicologists try to explain the phenomenon of pitch purely on the basis of Ohm's law, i.e. spectral information processing in the cochlea. This is certainly due to the fact that Ohm's law is relatively simple, while the processing mechanisms involved in the analysis of pitch are much more complex than had ever been imagined (see Chapters 7–9).

3.3   Hermann von Helmholtz

Hermann Helmholtz (Fig. 3.4) was born in 1821 in Potsdam near Berlin, the son of a teacher. As a young man he adored studying physics but was persuaded by his father to

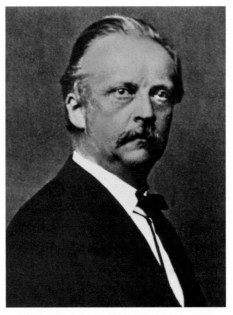

Fig. 3.4   Hermann von Helmholtz (1821–1894). His scientific work went far beyond the field of acoustics and hearing. His numerous discoveries and inventions made him one of the most influential and prestigious German scientists of his time (portrait by Ludwig Knaus, 1881, Alte Nationalgalerie, Berlin).

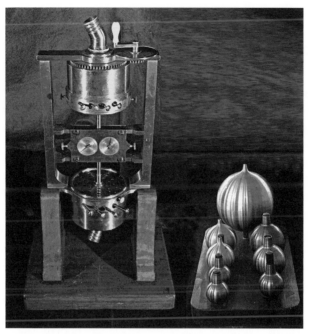

Fig. 3.5   Helmholtz's siren (left) and resonance spheres (right) can still be seen at the University of Heidelberg (photo by M. Camargo, Darmstadt University of Technology).

study medicine instead. After several years (1843–1848) as a medical officer in the royal regiment he was appointed as a professor of physiology in Berlin, Königsberg and Bonn.

Here, in 1851, 12 years after the Ohm–Seebeck dispute, the young physicist and physiologist started to devote much of his time to theories and experiments on hearing. He not only worked with his piano and various other musical instruments, but also experimented with all sorts of less musical apparatus – tuning forks, empty glass bottles, sirens and resonance spheres, subsequently known as 'Helmholtz spheres' (Fig. 3.5).

Helmholtz's experimental expertise was not limited to the field of acoustics and hearing; he made important contributions to many other scientific areas, including optics, vision, nerve and muscle physiology, electrodynamics and mathematics, and also to philosophy. His many discoveries and inventions – one of which, the ophthalmoscope, is still in use today – contributed to his fame as one of the most influential and prestigious German scientists of his time. Helmholtz received many honours during his lifetime and, in 1882, the German emperor officially granted him the noble title of Hermann 'von' Helmholtz.

3.4   A mechanical basis of pitch?

3.4.1   The 'cochlear piano'

In 1863 Helmholtz published his monumental book *On the Sensations of Tone as a Physiological Basis for the Theory of Music* (Helmholtz, 1863, 1954). It was based to a large extent on his own observations and experiments and his, for that time, revolutionary theories about musical perception and the mechanisms of sound production and sensation.

Twelve years earlier, in 1851, an Italian anatomist, Marchese Alfonso Corti (1822–1876), had employed his powerful new microscope to investigate the structure of the inner ear, the cochlea. Looking inside the cochlea he had observed the basilar membrane and the diverse structures resting on it – now known as the organ of Corti (see Box 6.2). Corti was the first to describe and make drawings of the tiny ciliated sensory hair cells ('Corti's cells'). It didn't take long for Helmholtz to realize the importance of these findings. Based on Corti's observations he developed a theory that also incorporated Ohm's acoustic law as well as some physiological ideas from his former mentor, Johannes Müller (1801–1858).

In his famous theory of resonance, Helmholtz postulated that the stretched fibres of Corti's basilar membrane function like the strings of a piano, an idea that was later illustrated by the – somewhat amusing – picture of a snail keyboard (the cochlear piano). He believed that the mechanical properties – length, thickness, elasticity and tension – of the fibres would allow them to resonate like piano strings at certain frequencies. Only the right frequency would be able to activate a certain fibre of the basilar membrane, which in turn would stimulate a certain nerve fibre. In his own words: 'Every simple tone of determinate pitch will be felt only by certain nerve fibres, and simple tones of different pitch will excite different fibres' (Helmholtz, 1954: p. 147).

3.4.2   Place and resonance

Helmholtz's assumption that different nerve fibres within the auditory nerve must code different pitches sprang from Müller's doctrine concerning the 'specific energy' of senses. This idea had originally been limited to different sensations across the five main sensory modalities (hearing, vision, taste, smell, touch), but Helmholtz elaborated and extended the idea to also include sensory sub-modalities. Accordingly, specific sensory information, such as colour or pitch, should be coded by a specific sensory channel. Today, this idea is often referred to as the 'labelled-line' principle.

Helmholtz also drew on the work of Thomas Young (1773–1829), an English physicist whose theory on vision had previously been given little attention. Helmholtz revived and advanced Young's ideas and incorporated them into the – still famous – Young–Helmholtz theory of colour vision. It suggests that qualitative differences in colour sensations may be reduced to differences in the nerve fibres that receive the sensations; Helmholtz argued that the same must be true for both differences in pitch and qualities of tones (timbre) in the hearing system.

The resonance aspect of Helmholtz's theory is complemented by his 'place principle'. This principle postulates that a certain pitch is signalled at a certain *place* on the basilar membrane because the fibres of the basilar membrane – again, just like the strings in a piano – are short at one end (at the base) and long at the other end (at the apex). The place principle gained some support in the first half of the twentieth century, when Georg von Békésy finally discovered travelling waves on the basilar membrane (see Fig. 6.4). Békésy could also show that pure tones elicit maximal wave amplitudes at frequency-dependent locations of the membrane (see Chapter 6). Consequently, many modern textbooks on hearing mechanisms still favour Helmholtz's place principle, thereby ignoring the fact that pitch is not a simple perceptual equivalent of frequency (see also Chapters 2 and 4).

Helmholtz had successfully drawn together several key ideas and discoveries and consolidated them into a mechanical theory of pitch based on selective resonance. His theory attracted considerable attention and was generally well accepted. It was only later that it became clear that the transverse fibres of the basilar membrane are not under suitable tension and therefore are unable to oscillate independently from each other, as Helmholtz had postulated. Moreover, although Békésy's travelling waves could be taken as evidence for Helmholtz's place principle, the wave mechanism was certainly quite different from Helmholtz's resonating fibres (see Chapter 4).

More than 100 years later it turned out that the place principle was only right to a certain extent. Depending on its loudness, a certain frequency may excite a more or less large extent of the basilar membrane (see Section 6.2). Moreover, as already discussed in the previous chapter, the same pitch may be perceived in completely different frequency ranges (e.g. the formant regions in Fig. 2.9). Alternatively, different pitches may be coded by different signal periodicities in one and the same frequency region and there-fore also at the same place on the basilar membrane. Obviously, Helmholtz's place theory cannot adequately explain pitch perception. As the following chapters will show, a correct explanation has to take account of temporal information coding in the auditory nerve and the central auditory system.

3.5   Combination tones and the missing fundamental

Helmholtz was convinced that, in accordance with Ohm's acoustical law, the cochlea performs a Fourier analysis and each tuned resonator which contributes to this analysis produces a certain sensation of pitch: 'One place, one pitch.' He claimed that each harmonic should have a pitch of its own, although inaudible in the presence of a strong fundamental frequency. In contrast to Seebeck, he believed that it is the fundamental alone that determines the pitch of the sound, while the other harmonics just have an impact on its timbre. As a consequence, he had to give up the idea of the periodic complex tone as a single entity, an idea that had been essential to researchers and philosophers for over two millennia, since the time of Pythagoras.

Long before Helmholtz, musicians and scientists were aware that a combination of frequencies can create a new pitch that differs from its constituents. A well-known example is the Tartini pitch (or Tartini tone), named after one of its discoverers, the Italian violinist and musical theorist Giuseppe Tartini (1692–1770). Two simultaneous tones with different pitches may elicit the percept of a third pitch with a frequency that corresponds to their frequency difference (see, for example, Fig. 2.5).

Helmholtz claimed that he had found a possible explanation for this effect on the basis of combination tones. Such non-linear distortion products result when a system – such as the eardrum – does not respond proportionally to signal amplitude, but instead responds, to a certain extent, also proportionally to its square. Helmholtz was able to generate strong tones using tuning forks and amplify them with his resonance spheres (Fig. 3.5). In this way he could actually demonstrate that the ear generates weak but audible combination tones when stimulated with two or more loud, simultaneous tones. His explanation was that the eardrum generated an actual physical component.

Nowadays it is clear that tone combinations, if loud enough, may in fact generate very weak combination tones, although only in the inner ear. Nevertheless, the important aspect of Helmholtz's conclusion remains true: combination tones are real physical vibrations which stimulate the ear in just the same way as external sound sources.

Although Helmholtz admitted that Seebeck may have heard the pitch of an absent fundamental, he claimed that it must have been the result of non-linear distortion, either produced at the eardrum or else, to a certain extent, already present in Seebeck's siren. He was convinced that Ohm's acoustical law holds: all audible tones, including those heard by Seebeck, correspond to the sinusoidal oscillations of real tones generated either outside or inside the ear. Altogether, in contrast to Seebeck, Helmholtz decided to reject the ear as a reliable judge of the nature of tones that faithfully represent the acoustic world. As a consequence, he also dismissed Seebeck's work, even casting doubt on the reliability of his observations (Schouten, 1970). In fact, Helmholtz's erroneous rejection of Seebeck's fundamental discovery is only the first case of a missing fundamental percept being misinterpreted as a distortion product.

3.6   A mechanical basis of harmony?

As early as the seventeenth century some scientists, such as Galileo Galilei (1564–1642), had discovered that the length of a string is not a unique determinant of pitch. While string lengths provide simple numerical ratios for harmonically related tones (Fig. 1.4), their gauges (thickness), for example, have to be squared to express pitch relationships (4:1 instead of 2:1 for an octave; 9:4 for a fifth). Perhaps even worse, if the frequency of vibration is considered instead of string length, then the harmonic ratios of octaves are reversed from 2:1 to 1:2. This shed some doubt on Pythagoras' ideas about the importance of simple integer number relationships for harmony; how could it be that the relationship of simple integers to harmonic perception is a 'universal law' if rather than the length of a string, its vibration frequency, or perhaps another string parameter, is crucial for pitch perception?

We will see that Seebeck was right and that the most relevant parameter is in fact the period of the sound. Period and frequency are only equivalent in cases where the wave repeats itself long enough so one can actually measure a frequency by counting enough repetitions. In natural sounds, as in music and speech, the period, and thus the pitch we perceive, may rapidly change; a frequency measurement will therefore only provide an average value. In order to fully account for our perception, frequency has to be replaced by a different parameter, such as the 'momentary frequency' (measured over a short interval) or, even better, the sound period.

At the beginning of his book about the sensation of tone, Helmholtz addresses the 'wonderful and meaningful mystery' of the relation of 'integers and musical consonance' that the 'Pythagoreans related to the harmony of the spheres' (Helmholtz, 1863: p. 27). In an attempt to solve this mystery, Helmholtz formed his own theory of consonance. He stated that our perception of musical harmony or consonance results from the absence of dissonance. Such dissonance or roughness results when tones are superposed that differ more or less in frequency (see Fig. 2.5).

In order to characterize the dissonance between two simultaneous musical tones, Helmholtz had to make particular reference to their harmonics. If there is a deviation of the fundamental frequencies of two tones ($f_1 - f_2$), the beat frequency between the nth harmonics of the tones ($n \cdot (f_1 - f_2)$) increases proportionally to their order number n. As a result, the roughness or dissonance of the tones depends on the numbers and frequency differences as well as on the amplitudes of their harmonics.

Using a rather arbitrary definition as a measure of the resulting overall dissonance of all relevant harmonics, Helmholtz was able to sum up the roughness for different tone pairs. In this way he could come up with a ranking list for harmonic relationships – from octaves to half-tones – which was in fact in line with Pythagoras' tetrakys and integer law (see Fig. 1.5). In spite of this remarkable although not quite accidental correspondence, Helmholtz had to realize that his explanation of consonance by minimal dissonance was quite different from the Pythagorean idea of the 'harmony of the inner and outer world'. In 1869, during an introductory talk at the Natural Science Congress in Innsbruck, he even rejected Pythagoras' fundamental concept, claiming it had been 'cruelly smashed to pieces' (Rieger, 2006).

In contrast to Helmholtz, contemporary musical experts clearly recognized that the pleasures of music, such as the wonder of an enchanting melody, could not be explained simply by the absence of roughness in certain tone combinations, and therefore criticized Helmholtz's theory vigorously. Among these was Hugo Riemann (1849–1919), an important German music theorist who rejected not only Helmholtz's explanation of harmony, but also his explanation of minor chords as 'clouded consonance' (Rieger, 2006). According to Riemann, the minor chord represents a mirror-symmetric complement of the major chord, a concept that is in line with conclusions about harmonic perception derived from the neuronal periodicity analysis (see Chapter 11).

3.7   Helmholtz's influence on music

In an attempt to analyse the essential basis of music – the melody – Helmholtz tried to explain the deficiencies in his consonance theory (Helmholtz, 1863: p. 299). First, he claimed that our ear creates harmonic overtones even when listening to pure tones, and second, that we are able to memorize those combinations of complex tones which would create less dissonant sounds. Thus, Helmholtz had effectively reduced the 'great Pythagorean mystery' to the imperfect processing capabilities of our ear, in combination with auditory memory.

It seems that, especially in the twentieth century, Helmholtz's theory of tone perception resulted in an elevated appreciation of the timbre of musical sounds versus harmony and melody. Harmony and melody were increasingly considered to be somewhat questionable ingredients, arising merely as a consequence of individual and cultural experience and memory. Up to the present time, many musicians seem to have accepted this concept of the dominance and importance of timbre. Helmholtz's influence on composers like Leos Janacek, Paul Hindemith, Georg Ives and Arnold Schönberg is well documented in the music–scientific literature (Rieger, 2006).

4 The pitch puzzle

4.1 The telephone theory

Although a broadband harmonic sound, for example a human vowel (see Figs. 2.8, 2.9), activates many sensory cells along the basilar membrane, it is typically perceived as an entirety and has just a single pitch. We neither hear the rapid amplitude fluctuations, due to its periodic envelope, nor realize that it is composed of a fundamental frequency and perhaps dozens of harmonics, which all have quite different pitches when heard separately. Helmholtz was able to single out individual harmonics of tones by means of his spherical resonators (see Fig. 3.5), but he could not explain the fusion of these harmonics into single tones with just one pitch. This puzzle remained a challenge for scientists from the nineteenth century to the present time (Stumpf, 1890; Ebeling, 2008).

To overcome this, and other drawbacks of Helmholtz's resonance theory, the Scottish physiologist William Rutherford (1839–1899) proposed an alternative idea. In 1886, in a lecture to the British Association for the Advancement of Science in Birmingham, he postulated that the ear functions like a telephone, the pioneering device that had been invented only ten years earlier by Alexander Graham Bell (1847–1922). While Helmholtz had compared the basilar membrane to a piano, Rutherford, on the basis of his own anatomical investigations, had come to the conclusion that the basilar membrane must vibrate as a whole, just like the membrane of a telephone.

Consequently, the sensory cells of the inner ear should pick up the mechanical sound vibrations, transform them into electrical currents and transmit the resulting signal via 'cables' (the auditory nerve fibres) to the receiver (the brain). As a result, the essential auditory information would be coded exclusively in the time domain and the nerve fibres would have to transfer merely temporal signals to the brain for further temporal processing.

A potential problem with this theory, however, is that it would require a very high transmission rate to the brain. Helmholtz had measured the velocity of nerve impulses in frogs and his results suggested that rates of acoustic information transmission in the auditory nerve, although quite high, must be limited to frequencies below about 1 kHz. Yet it was obvious that much higher frequencies than this are necessary for the understanding of speech (−3 kHz) and the full enjoyment of music (−15 kHz). Unfortunately, Rutherford could not answer the question of how his cochlear telephone might transfer these higher frequencies to the brain. As always when a new theory is developed, more questions arise than can be answered.

Nevertheless, Rutherford's telephone model was the first serious challenge to Helmholtz's theory of resonance, and it has in fact turned out – a century later – to contain elements of truth and to have significant medical relevance. Nowadays, several hundreds of thousands of deaf people all over the world make use of a telephone-like electronic device known as a cochlear implant. Electromagnetic transduction via coils implanted behind their ears and an electrode in their ear that transfers signals to the auditory nerve allow these patients to hear, perhaps for the first time in their life. Many patients are indeed able to even follow conversations on the telephone, when there is no possibility for additional lip-reading.

Some early versions of this medical wonder transferred signals successfully to just a single electrode channel, thereby disregarding cochlear place information completely (Hochmair and Hochmair, 1986). This proved beyond all doubt that our brain can process speech signals, even when nothing more than temporal information is available. Modern cochlear implants utilize spectro-temporal coding strategies with several electrodes along the basilar membrane. Usually, after sufficient training, these implants make speech comprehensible for many patients and music often becomes enjoyable.

4.2   'The Residue Revisited'

Even after the discovery of travelling waves by Békésy and the subsequent refutation of the resonance model, Helmholtz's place principle of cochlear frequency analysis dominated the field. Although over the years researchers increasingly felt that it might be too simple a solution for a complex problem, it wasn't until the summer of 1969 that a symposium with the title 'Frequency Analysis and Periodicity Detection in Hearing' was finally held in Driebergen (Netherlands). Since its main purpose was to discuss the continuing controversy about a spectral versus a temporal origin of pitch, several attempts to solve the pitch problem were presented by leading scientists. Most importantly for the present book, the Dutch biophysicist Jan Frederik Schouten (Fig. 4.1) gave a remarkable talk entitled 'The Residue Revisited' (Schouten, 1970), in which he summarized a series of papers, the first of which had been published almost 30 years earlier (Schouten, 1938; Schouten et al., 1962). Schouten emphasized the limits of Helmholtz's place principle and reintroduced Seebeck's idea of the 'missing fundamental': the periodic signal envelope of a complex tone, not the fundamental, is essential for the generation of a certain pitch. This is true for all kinds of signals that have no fundamental component, such as amplitude-modulated sine waves with just three frequency components (AM signals, Figs. 2.6, 4.4). Schouten, therefore, introduced the concept of a 'residue' that encompasses the pitch of the 'missing fundamental' of harmonic sounds as well as that of AM signals.

At the symposium in Driebergen, Schouten interpreted the residue as the tonal sensation of the superimposed higher-frequency components of a periodic sound and postulated 'a set of parallel pitch extractors' that analyse the period of the signals in 'narrow frequency channels' (Schouten, 1970). As an example, he showed how a series of clicks with 5 ms intervals would be represented in the cochlea (Fig. 4.2). Schouten's

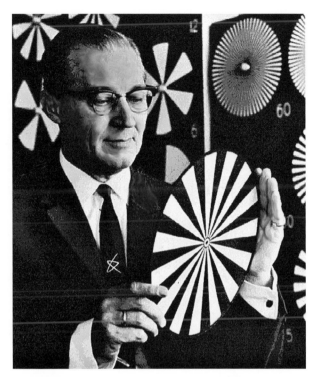

Fig. 4.1   Jan Frederik Schouten (1910–1980), biophysicist and professor at the Technical University Eindhoven (Netherlands), invented an electro-optical siren which allowed him to translate optical signals into periodical sound signals and to address with high precision the problem of the 'missing fundamental' (the picture shows Schouten with components of his optical sirens; by courtesy of Don Bouwhuis, Technical University Eindhoven).

idea was that the auditory nerve should code temporal as well as spectral information about the spatial activation of the sensory cells in the cochlea. The spectral information along the basilar membrane is essential for the timbre of a sound and corresponds to a (quasi-)Fourier spectrum of the signal with a limited frequency resolution (Fig. 4.2b), while the temporal information is essential for the pitch of a sound and codes the periodicities and interval patterns of the filtered waveforms (Fig. 4.2c).

Due to the limited resolving power of the cochlear filter, one area of the basilar membrane may respond to several frequency components of a harmonic sound. Because the difference frequency of adjacent harmonics is equal to the fundamental frequency, the envelope periods of the responses (filtered waveforms, Fig. 4.2c) are equal to the period of the whole signal (and to the period of the fundamental frequency alone). According to Schouten this temporal filter effect explains why the pitch of each filtered wave, when presented in isolation, is equal to the pitch of the whole signal and to the – perhaps even missing – fundamental frequency.

Here, we should remember that Helmholtz had dismissed Seebeck's missing fundamental as being an artefact due to distortion products (Section 3.5). Nowadays it is well

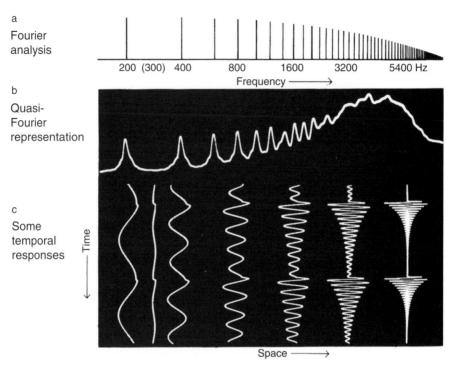

a
Fourier
analysis

200 (300) 400   800   1600   3200   5400 Hz
Frequency ⟶

b
Quasi-
Fourier
representation

c
Some
temporal
responses

⟵ Time

Space ⟶

Figure 4.2   (a) A Fourier analysis of a periodic signal (clicks with a period of 5 ms) reveals its harmonics. (b) The excitation pattern evoked by this signal on the basilar membrane corresponds to a quasi-Fourier spectrum. (c) The figure shows short segments of the responses on the basilar membrane at regular frequency distances. All response envelopes (but not the resolved second harmonic) have the same period as the fundamental frequency. Therefore they elicit the same (residual) pitch when presented individually (modified from Schouten, 1970).

known that under normal conditions and in healthy ears such distortions are generally quite weak (Zwicker and Feldtkeller, 1967). Furthermore, with the advent of electronic equipment – for example, the electro-optical siren invented by Schouten – it became possible to perform controlled psychophysical experiments by synthesizing complex acoustic signals with high precision and reproducibility.

Moreover, modern techniques allow one to exclude distortion tones as possible sources of the residual pitch of high-frequency sounds. By adding a loud-enough masking noise in the low-frequency range (Fig. 4.3), all possible distortion tones can be drowned out while the pitch of the missing fundamental, or residual pitch, remains perceivable (Licklider, 1951). This finding proved at the same time that Helmholtz's 'place principle' cannot explain the residual pitch: although the residuum is a low pitch, it is not elicited in the corresponding low, but in a higher-frequency region of the basilar membrane.

In summary, Schouten's discovery of the residue supported Seebeck's assumption that the harmonics of a complex sound contribute to the percept of its pitch. But Schouten also realized that the high-frequency components of harmonic sounds do not just

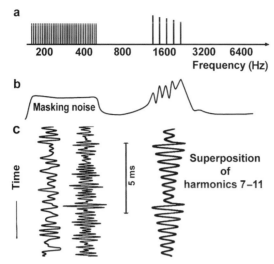

a

200   400   800   1600   3200 6400
Frequency (Hz)

b

Masking noise

c

Time

5 ms

Superposition
of
harmonics 7–11

Fig. 4.3   **(a)** The Fourier spectrum of a narrowband signal (modified from Fig. 4.2a) and of an additional low-frequency masking noise that excludes distortion products as a possible cause of the residual pitch. **(b)** The corresponding excitation pattern on the basilar membrane. **(c)** The periodic response on the basilar membrane that elicits the residual pitch together with the response to the masking noise. In such experiments the low residual pitch of this signal is clearly audible, in spite of the fact that the low-frequency noise masks all possible low-frequency distortion products.

somehow enhance the pitch of their fundamental frequency; instead, they elicit a totally new percept, the residue, with the same pitch but a different timbre.

4.3   The 'dominance region'

Although spectral filtering improves along the frequency axis of the cochlea (see Fig. 6.6), the spectral resolution of harmonic sounds on the basilar membrane is high for low harmonics and decreases with frequency (Fig. 4.2b). As a result of the increasing superposition of harmonics along the logarithmic cochlear axis (from left to right in Fig. 4.2c), the temporal modulation boosts with frequency and is most pronounced in the high-frequency region; it is weak or even absent for low harmonics (Fig. 4.2c). According to Schouten's periodicity theory, the pitch should therefore be more salient for high harmonics. However, much to his surprise, this is not the case. Instead, it could be demonstrated that there is a 'dominance region' for pitch extraction. It depends on the fundamental frequency of a harmonic sound and is located in the frequency region around the fourth harmonic, that is, the most salient periodicity pitch arises in this relatively low-frequency area (Ritsma, 1967; Schouten, 1970).

The existence of the dominance region indicated that Schouten's theory could not explain all relevant aspects of pitch perception; obviously, something was still missing. As we will see in Chapter 9, pitch processing requires the simultaneous coding and processing of spectrally resolved as well as unresolved harmonics by specialized neurons in the auditory brainstem (Langner, 1988).

4.4   The pitch shift

Schouten's original hypothesis was that the pitch of a sound signal is constant as long as the period of its envelope remains constant. However, when he and his co-workers introduced amplitude-modulated sine waves (AM signals) as test signals it turned out that this prediction did not hold: AM signals could have quite different pitches even when they had the same envelope period (Figs. 4.4, 4.5; Schouten *et al.*, 1962; Ritsma, 1970).

In the crucial experiments, in which Schouten described what is now called the 'first effect of pitch shift', listeners compared the pitch of an AM signal with that of a

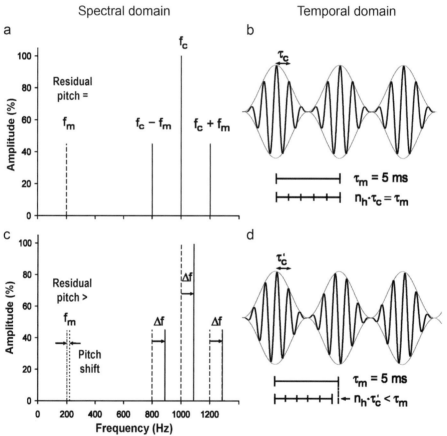

Fig. 4.4   **(a)** The spectrum of a harmonic AM signal (modulation frequency $f_m = 200$ Hz) is composed of the carrier frequency ($f_c = 1$ kHz), a lower and an upper sideband ($f_l = f_c - f_m$ and $f_u = f_c + f_m$). Note that the frequency f_m is not a physical component of the AM signal. **(b)** The modulation frequency is visible as the envelope of the signal waveform (thin line). The intervals below the waveform indicate that the modulation period τ_m corresponds to five carrier periods. The residual pitch equals the pitch of the modulation frequency (dashed line in **(a)**). **(c)** When the carrier is shifted by Δf and the AM signal becomes inharmonic, the modulation period becomes larger than five periods of the carrier and the residual pitch increases (dashed line in **(c)**).

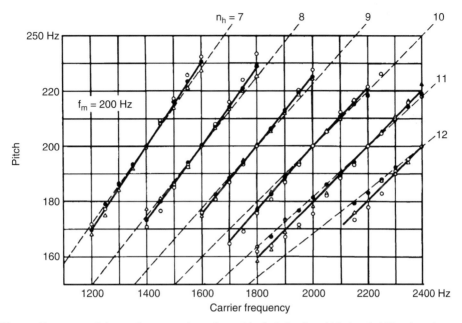

Fig. 4.5   Contrary to Schouten's expectations, the residual pitch of an AM signal shifts when the carrier frequency is varied around a centre ($f_c = 1200$–2400 Hz; $f_m = $ constant $= 200$ Hz; $n_h = 7$–12, three subjects). To a first approximation the resulting pitch corresponds to a subharmonic of the carrier frequency (f_c/n_h, dashed lines), close – but not equal – to the pitch of the constant modulation frequency. This relationship has been called the 'first effect of pitch shift'. However, the actually percepts (bold lines) deviated slightly, but consistently, from this approximation. The discrepancy was called the 'second effect of pitch shift' (Schouten *et al.*, 1962, slightly modified).

harmonic sound (Fig. 4.5). According to Schouten the results 'killed two birds with one stone' (Schouten, 1970): the pitch of AM signals is neither defined just by their temporal envelopes nor by their spectral compositions.

An AM signal with the modulation frequency f_m is composed of a carrier frequency f_c and two additional sidebands ($f_l = f_c - f_m$ and $f_u = f_c + f_m$; Fig. 4.4a). It is harmonic if the relation of its carrier f_c to f_m is given by an integer number, the harmonic ratio n_h ($= f_c/f_m$). Its envelope (thin line in Fig. 4.4b) is defined by the modulation frequency, but it does not contain a spectral component with that frequency (Fig. 4.4a). Nevertheless, Schouten found that its residual pitch P_r is always close to the pitch P_m of the modulation frequency f_m, these being equal in the harmonic case.

However, for inharmonic AM signals, when the carrier is shifted by a small amount Δf_c, the perceived pitch P_r deviates slightly, but systematically, from P_m (Fig. 4.4c, d) and a better approximation may be obtained from a subharmonic of the carrier frequency (P_r ($= f_c/n_h$). The fact that the pitch shifts in this case by about ΔP_r ($= \Delta f_c/n_h$) is called the 'first effect of pitch shift' (dashed line in Fig. 4.5). Although the 'first effect' shows that the modulation period does not exactly define the pitch of (inharmonic) AM signals, Schouten maintained that the solution to this pitch puzzle must be nevertheless a 'form of periodicity detection in the time domain' (Schouten, 1970). He was convinced that there must be 'temporal pitch extractors' in the brain and, moreover, that pitch sensation does not arise from two entirely different mechanisms, one for pure tones – the cochlear analysis – and one for complex tones – the neuronal analysis in the brain.

But this was still not the end of the pitch puzzle story. Sixteen years after Schouten's discovery, one of his students, Edward de Boer, repeated his experiments (de Boer, 1956). He confirmed his discovery, but he also realized that, when looked at more closely, the observed pitch values for non-harmonic AM signals deviated slightly but systematically from the values predicted by Schouten.

As verified by Schouten and his co-workers (Schouten *et al.*, 1962; Ritsma, 1970), there was indeed a small but systematic deviation from Schouten's prediction, which they named 'the second effect of pitch shift' (Fig. 4.5). Various spectral and temporal models have been developed since that time – including the ones presented in Chapter 9 of this book – which aimed at a possible solution of the pitch puzzle.

4.5   Spectral coding

Since the time of Seebeck it has become more and more clear that a low pitch (in a range that is particularly relevant for speech and music) may be perceived even when a sound is only composed of high frequencies. Obviously, our brain must be able to extract the residual pitch or the pitch of the missing fundamental from spectral or temporal features of these high frequencies, or perhaps from both.

As we have seen, an obvious temporal feature of a pitched signal is its envelope. Harmonic sounds with the same envelope period will also have the same pitch, quite independently of the details of their spectra. The first effect of pitch shift, however, undermined the role of the envelope as a solution for the pitch puzzle, because it showed that the pitch of inharmonic sounds may change even when their envelope period is kept constant. Moreover, the second effect of pitch shift challenged the possibility that the residual pitch is simply given by a subharmonic of the AM-carrier frequency.

Several theorists attempted to solve this puzzle; a few years after the symposium in Driebergen, different versions of so-called *pattern-recognition* models or simply 'pattern models' of pitch perception were published by Ernst Terhardt (1972a, 1972b), Julius Goldstein (1973) and Frederic L. Wightman (1973). All three of these, still popular, pattern models are based on the assumption that, in order to derive the periodicity pitch, our brain analyses the complex spatial activation pattern on the basilar membrane that represents the sound spectrum. As one would expect, the models differ in some respects. For instance, Goldstein's model postulates that the spectral information provided by the cochlea is initially enhanced by temporal coding. Nevertheless, in essence each of the models assumes that the central auditory system performs a kind of correlation analysis in the spectral domain.

One of the problems with pattern models is that they rely on the spectral resolution of signals on the basilar membrane. Therefore, the question arises of whether the components of periodic signals are indeed sufficiently resolved in all cases where a periodicity pitch can be heard. The lower components of a harmonic signal, at least, may be clearly resolved when amplified by Helmholtz resonators (Fig. 3.5). Modern psychophysics supports Helmholtz's observation that harmonics below about the twelfth order are partially resolved and may be perceived under appropriate conditions (Moore *et al.*, 2006). However, the resolving power of our hearing system does not exclude the interference of adjacent harmonic frequency components, at least to a certain extent (Fig. 4.2c). In fact, harmonics above the seventh order interfere considerably already (Moore *et al.*, 2006). In addition, and unfortunately for the pattern models, periodicity pitch also exists in the range of clearly unresolved harmonics above the twelfth harmonic (Kaernbach and Bering, 2001), a fact which these models completely fail to explain.

4.6   Temporal coding

At the time when the pattern models were formulated, it was already clear that our brain is able to temporally analyse acoustic signals with high precision. The most convincing evidence comes from our remarkable ability to localize sound sources that are separated in the horizontal plane by as little as one degree (Zwicker and Feldtkeller, 1967). While for frequencies above about 1000 Hz we can make use of the shadow effect of our head, below that frequency this effect is small and temporal processing becomes the only possible solution. This allows us to localize sound sources that reach our ears with a time difference of only 10 μs (Jeffress, 1948).

In the last 30 years it has become increasingly clear that auditory nerve fibres code temporal information with a precision that is adequate for pitch analysis (see Chapters 6 and 7). Consequently, the fact that a periodicity pitch (residue) can be perceived not only from low-order resolved harmonics but also from high-order unresolved harmonics has led to a variety of models (see Chapter 9) which, in contrast to the pattern models, include temporal information from both low and high harmonics (Moore, 1982; Plack and Oxenham, 2005).

If our hearing system does indeed analyse temporal intervals to determine the pitch of periodic signals, the signal parameters of pitch experiments as well as the measured pitch values should be expressed in the temporal domain, i.e. as intervals or periods instead of frequencies (Langner, 1981, 1992, 1997). Therefore, in Fig. 4.6 Schouten's pitch data (Fig. 4.5) were analysed again by a linear regression analysis using temporal coordinates: the carrier frequencies f_c of the AM signals were replaced by the carrier period τ_c (= $1/f_c$) and the measured pitch values P by the pitch period τ_p (= $1/P$). The data points in Fig. 4.6a indicate the average slopes (n) of the perceived pitch shifts in the temporal domain ($\tau_p = n \cdot \tau_c - \tau_k$). According to Schouten's first effect of pitch shift, the points should align along the dashed line corresponding to the harmonic ratios (n = n_h) and the axis intercepts (τ_k) of the linear fits of the pitch shifts would be zero. However, due to the second effect of pitch shift the slopes are slightly larger than the harmonic ratio (n > n_h) while the intercepts are larger than zero and range between 0.4 and 0.8 ms.

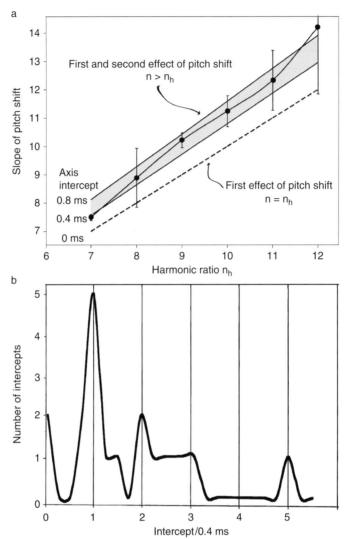

Fig. 4.6 (a) In contrast to Schouten's interpretation of the pitch data in the *spectral* domain (see Fig. 4.5), the figure presents the results of a linear regression analysis of the same data in the *temporal* domain, i.e. the (residual) pitch *period* τ_p is related to the carrier *period* τ_c of the AM signal. The data points indicate the corresponding average slopes (n) of the observed pitch shifts. According to Schouten's first effect the pitch should be a subharmonic of the carrier frequency and the slopes would align along the dashed line ($n = n_h$ = harmonic ratio, $\tau_p = n_h \cdot \tau_c$). However, due to the second effect the slopes of the pitch shifts are somewhat larger than the harmonic ratio ($n > n_h$) while the intercepts (τ_k) of the regression analysis range between 0.4 and 0.8 ms ($\tau_p = n \cdot \tau_c - \tau_k$; see also Fig. 4.4d). **(b)** A detailed analysis reveals that the axis intercepts cluster at certain integer multiples of 0.4 ms.

A closer look reveals that the slopes of the pitch curves vary not only from subject to subject, but also for the upper and lower half of each individual curve. A corresponding linear regression analysis results in axis intercepts that cluster at certain small integer multiples of an interval of 0.4 ms (Fig. 4.6b). Note that the same time constant has already appeared in Fig. 2.10, as corner points of the vowel triangle. In the next chapter further evidence for this perceptual constant is presented, and in Chapter 9 this effect will be explained on the basis of a neuronal correlation analysis including intrinsic oscillation periods that are also integer multiples of 0.4 ms.

5 The auditory time constant

'Panpipes and flutes obey the same law.'

From a Chinese fairy tale by Tung Chou Li Kuo Tse, about 1600

(Hornbostel, 1928)

5.1   A quantum effect of pitch shift

In the previous chapter the pitch shifts measured by Schouten were analysed by employing periods instead of frequencies for the signal as well as for the perceived pitches. The resulting linear approximations of the pitch shifts in the time domain revealed auditory mechanisms which are obviously able to extract integer multiples of the period of the carrier.

Moreover, it also provided evidence for perceptual time constants that are not related to the periods of the signal. Actually, these constants may be put down to just one, since they are also integer multiples, not of a signal period but of an intrinsic auditory time constant of 0.40 ms. It will be shown in the following that this value is characteristic for the hearing system and seems to function as a kind of auditory benchmark, not only in human speech and music, but also in animal communication (see also Chapter 9).

The presumed auditory time constant becomes even more plausible by another perceptual effect that may be called the 'third' or 'quantal effect of pitch shift' (Langner, 1981, 1983). When experimental subjects compared the residual pitch of an AM signal (see Fig. 4.4) with that of a pure tone, they frequently reported that, although they heard the pitch increase with the carrier frequency f_c, it did so not in a continuous, but in a staircase-like manner. The pitch steps were small but of equal size when measured in the time domain – that is, as temporal intervals.

As an example, Fig. 5.1 shows results from such measurements (Langner, 1981). Two subjects compared the pitch of an AM signal with varying carrier frequency to that of pure tones. Both subjects heard pitches that corresponded approximately to the sixth subharmonic of the carrier frequency, that is, the periods of the tones they selected for comparison matched up to six periods of the carrier. But when the periods of the pitch approached an integer multiple of 0.4 ms the subjects reported pitch percepts that corresponded to these intervals. Consequently, the pitch increased in steps of about 0.4 ms, as indicated by the step curves in Fig 5.1 (thin lines).

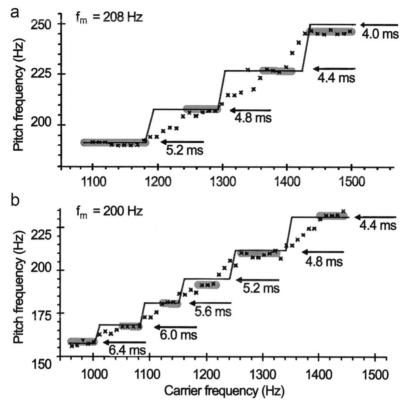

Fig. 5.1   When the carrier frequency of an AM signal is increased, the period of the perceived pitch tends to change in steps of about 0.4 ms. Corresponding results of experiments with two subjects **(a, b)** are shown (**a**: $f_c = 1100–1500$ Hz, $f_m = 208$ Hz; **b**: $f_c = 960–1440$ Hz, $f_m = 200$ Hz). If one takes these results together the preference for pitch periods that are multiples of 0.4 ms is highly significant (Gauss-test, 0.40 ms ± 0.03 ms, $p < 1\%$). The depicted staircases (thin lines) approximate the 'quantal pitch shift' (constant pitch ranges are labelled in grey). Note that in both cases the effect (grey labels) is more pronounced in the second half of the stairs where $6\tau_c < n \cdot 0.4$ ms **(a)**, or $< n \cdot 0.4$ ms–0.2 ms **(b)**. **(a)** In the centres of the stairs the carrier period τ_c fulfils exactly the condition $6\tau_c = n \cdot 0.4$ ms (n = 10–13). **(b)** In this case the condition is $6\tau_c = n \cdot 0.4$ ms–0.2 ms (n = 10–15). The difference of 0.2 ms may be explained by the fact that here the modulation period ($\tau_m = 5$ ms) is by 0.2 ms larger than in **(a)**.

The quantal pitch shift may be explained by the coincidence of neuronal responses that are phase-coupled, on the one hand, to the carrier and, on the other hand, to the modulation of an AM signal. Additional delays are introduced by synchronized intrinsic oscillations with periods that are multiples of 0.4 ms (see Chapter 9).

The oscillations obviously provide references or benchmarks for the definition of signal periods and – under certain conditions – they may dominate the pitch percept resulting in ranges of constant pitch and pitch steps. In Chapter 9 the oscillations are attributed to specialized neurons (chopper neurons) in the cochlear nucleus, the first centre of the central auditory system (for more details, see Chapter 6).

5.2   Pulling effect and absolute pitch

The described quantal pitch effect reminds one of the so-called 'pulling effect' of certain physical and biological oscillators. As a result of mutual synchronization, such oscillators may shift their resonance frequencies as if they were pulling each other. The first person who observed and described in detail such an effect was the Dutch physicist Christiaan Huygens in 1665. Much to his amazement, two of his pendulum clocks were able to mutually adjust their frequencies and synchronize them over a long time. Although an experienced scientist, he had a hard time finding out how they actually interact: not through the air, as he had first thought, but through the wooden wall to which they were attached (Bennett, 2002).

The pulling effect works only when two oscillators, like Huygens' clocks, have quite similar resonance frequencies. If one knows this frequency for one oscillator, the observation of the pulling effect allows one to conclude that the other oscillator must have the same frequency, that is, one oscillator may serve as a reference for the other. Therefore, an obvious conclusion from the auditory pulling effect (the quantal effect of pitch shift) is that our auditory system may have access to an intrinsic oscillation (Chapter 9) that can serve as an absolute temporal reference.

Most of us perceive pitch relatively. We recognize and memorize melodic and harmonic relationships of pitches instead of perceiving absolute pitch values. On the other hand, very few people have absolute or 'perfect' pitch (Ward, 1999). These people are able to identify pitches effortlessly and immediately and name them without the use of any external reference (Bachem, 1955). However, any kind of absolute measurement necessarily requires some kind of a reference. Consequently, for an absolute definition of pitch it seems indispensable that there is a temporal reference in the auditory system. That, in principle, all of us may have such an internal pitch reference at our disposal is indicated by the quantal pitch effect, and it is likely that the capability of absolute pitch is due to the same intrinsic temporal scale.

5.3   The auditory time constant in vowel formants

The auditory time constant of 0.4 ms does not only appear in sophisticated pitch experiments. As an example for a possible more extensive role of this perceptual constant, we have seen in Chapter 2 that the corners of the two-dimensional distribution of vowel formants in the formant plane may be related to integer multiples of 0.4 ms.

This is in line with a corresponding interpretation of the results of a classical study by Gordon E. Peterson and Harold L. Barney from the Bell Telephone Laboratories in Murray Hill, New Jersey in 1954 (Fig. 5.2). They showed that – for their selection of speakers from various regions of the United States – different vowels are represented in the plane of

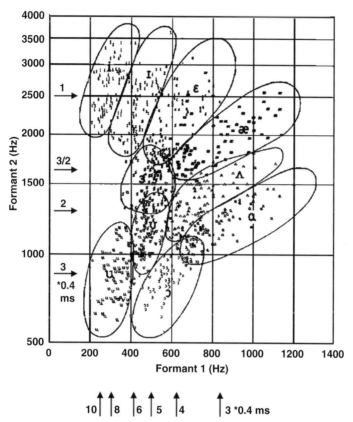

Fig. 5.2　The graphic shows the distribution of frequencies of the first and second formants for ten vowels pronounced by 33 men, 28 women and 15 children (modified from Peterson and Barney, 1952). The majority of the speakers spoke General American English with a broad regional sampling of the United States. As a result, the encircled areas of formant frequencies for single vowels are quite broad and partly overlapping. Nevertheless, the centres of these areas obviously correlate with certain frequencies (F_2: 2500, 1667 = 2 · 833, 1250, 833 Hz; F_1: 833, 625, 500, 417, 313 Hz); their periods are integer multiples (F_2: 1–3; F_1: 3–6, 8) of 0.4 ms, or – in three cases – 3/2 times 0.4 ms.

formants in areas that are mostly separated, but also quite broad and partly overlapping. As indicated by arrows (added to the original figure) both formants cluster around particular frequencies with the corresponding periods being integer multiples of 0.4 ms (for details see legend of Fig. 5.2). This result suggests that the supposed auditory time constant may also play a role in speech, especially for the generation and recognition of vowels.

One may wonder why the boundaries between vowels in Fig. 5.2 are not horizontal and vertical lines parallel to the coordinate axes, representing the formants F_1 and F_2. It is not quite clear why this is not the case, but for synthesized, simplified vowels such straight boundaries in the formant planes have already been shown (Chistovich and Lublinskaya, 1979.; Hose *et al.*, 1983). This suggests that – at least for such artificial vowels – the vowel categories are delineated by each formant 'separately'. More precisely, provided one formant of such a vowel,

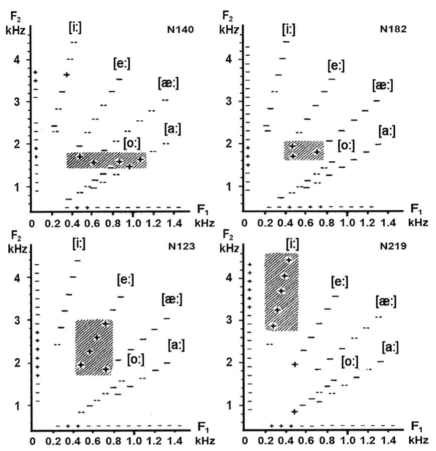

Fig. 5.3   Neurons in the auditory 'cortex' (Field L) of speech-trained mynah birds were found that respond selectively to human vowels. Above, the responses of four neurons to artificial vowels (composed of only six harmonics) are mapped in the plane of formants. Excitatory responses are indicated by '+' and inhibitory responses by '–' (in relation to the spontaneous activity of the neurons). The responses are simple combinations of the responses to the isolated formants F_1 and F_2 alone, as plotted along the axes (modified from Langner *et al.*, 1981).

e.g. F_2, is located in a certain frequency range, the other formant (F_1) alone determines which of several possible vowels may be perceived and several vowels may share the same boundary for F_1. The conclusion that recognition of (at least artificial) vowels relies on independent processing of the formants and a small number of critical frequencies with periods that are integer multiples of the auditory time constant of 0.4 ms.

This interpretation is supported by investigations of neurons in Field L, the analogue of the mammalian primary auditory cortex, in speech imitating mynah birds. About 10% of the examined neurons turned out to be selective to certain natural vowels (Langner *et al.*, 1981). By applying synthetic vowels as well as single formants this selectivity could be attributed to a convergence of multiple excitatory and inhibitory frequency channels on these neurons (Fig. 5.3). If one formant fell into an excitatory

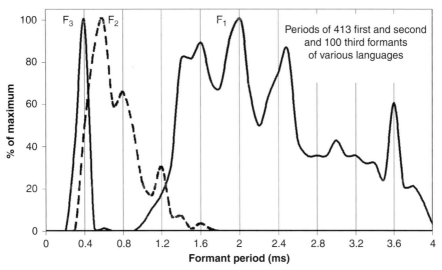

Fig. 5.4   The three curves show the distribution of the periods of formant frequencies as measured in vowels of 27 languages and 15 dialects of some of these languages. The maxima of the distributions indicate highly significant preferences for formant periods that are integer multiples of 0.40 ms ± 0.01 ms (Gauss-test: $p < 0.1\%$). Note that the distribution for F_2 has its main maximum at 0.6 ms, which may result from a frequency reduction (or period doubling: $2 \cdot 0.6$ ms = 1.2 ms).

frequency band (as indicated along the formant axes in Fig. 5.3), the second formant had to coincide also with an excitatory – or at least neutral – band for the complete vowel to produce a response. Furthermore, other vowels were rejected by such a neuron if one or both of their formants fell into inhibitory bands that suppressed all excitation.

This finding of an additive or subtractive interaction of formant responses may give rise to a simple hypothesis for the straight vowel boundaries as found in psychophysical experiments (see above). The vowel boundaries would be parallel to the formant axes because in vowel processing neurons the response to one formant may be suppressed or enhanced by the response to the other formant, but not significantly altered. The finding may also be taken as a hint that neuronal mechanisms in animals may be quite comparable to those in our brain.

Further support for the role of the auditory time constant of 0.4 ms in speech generation and recognition comes from the frequency distributions of the first three formants of human vowels. The data shown in Fig. 5.4 were obtained from hundreds of vowels from 27 languages and 15 dialects of some languages assembled from various sources on the internet (e.g. helsinki.fi/speechsciences, home.cc.umanitoba.ca, linguistics.ucla.edu, yorku.ca). Although the quality and reliability of the evaluated internet data are certainly quite variable, the result is nevertheless intriguing. In line with the conclusions based on the Peterson–Barney study (see above), each of the formant distributions has significant maxima at periods corresponding to integer multiples of 0.4 ms (for more details, see the legend of Fig. 5.4).

Finally, Fig. 5.5 shows that this correspondence may perhaps be extended to all known vowel categories. A typical language, such as English, contains about 11

		F_2							
1	2500	[i̯]	[i:]	[i]	[ɪ]	[ə]	[e]	[ɛ]	[ɛ:]
3/2	1667	-	[ʏ]	[y:]	[y]	[œ]	[3]	[e:]	[æ]
2	1250	-	-	[u:]	[ʊ]	[ø:]	[a:]	[ʌ]	[a]
3	833	-	-	-	[u]	[o]	[ɔ]	[o:]	-
[Hz]/[Hz]		250	278	313	357	417	500	625	833	F_1
		10	9	8	7	6	5	4	3

(left axis) $1/(F_2 \cdot 0.4\,ms)$

$1/(F_1 \cdot 0.4\,ms)$

Fig. 5.5   The table show all (25) possible standard vowel categories and indicates that they may be related to formant periods that are close to integer multiples of 0.4 ms (with the exception of 3/2; see also Fig. 5.2). Although there are significant variations of actual measurements, especially in different languages, the table suggests that there may be a one-to-one relationship between all possible vowel categories and the 0.4 ms matrix.

vowel categories, while there may be altogether about 25 different vowel categories if one considers all languages. Although the details about the formant frequencies may vary a lot, one may relate them more or less all to periods that are integer multiples of 0.40 ms (the exception of 1.5 was already discussed in the legend of Fig. 5.2). Note that Fig. 5.5 does not have any gaps; that is, all possible combinations of multiples of 0.40 ms may correspond to a particular vowel category. On the other hand, the boundaries of this correspondence indicate that F_2 should be larger than about 800 Hz and must also be larger than F_1 (by definition). Moreover, the lower boundary mostly indicates that F_1 must be well above the fundamental frequency of the vowels. These statements are complemented by the clear relation of the third formant to 0.4 ms (Fig. 5.4).

5.4   The auditory time constant in Chinese tone language

In 2007 I had the opportunity to give a talk about temporal processing in the auditory system in the laboratory of Diana Deutsch, professor of psychology at the University of California in San Diego. Diana Deutsch is very well known for her research on perception and memory for speech and music, and for her discovery of numerous stunning auditory illusions and paradoxes. At the time of my visit she was especially interested in the mystery of absolute (or perfect) pitch. She told me that this amazing capability to identify and name single tones seems to be abundant among speakers of tone languages, like Mandarin (Chinese) and Vietnamese, while it is quite rare among speakers of non-tone languages (Deutsch *et al.*, 2006). With my own hypothesis in mind, that absolute pitch must be somehow based on the auditory time constant, I asked what the pitch was of the speech probe she presented to me. Sure enough, the dominant pitch of this sample was 250 Hz, corresponding to a period of ten times 0.4 ms. This finding triggered my interest and research in this field: the question was whether this pitch value was a mere

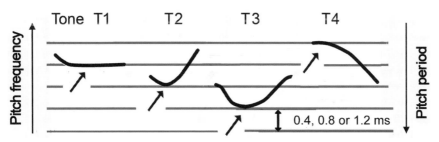

Fig. 5.6   The simplified scheme illustrates the pitch contours of the four so-called 'tones' of Mandarin, a Chinese tone language. The arrows point to segments of more or less constant pitch that tend to differ by 0.4, 0.8 or 1.2 ms (see Fig. 5.4). The standard deviations of the segments with constant pitches, used for the evaluation in Fig. 5.8, are below 5%, for T1 even below 1%.

coincidence or if the Chinese tone language indeed refers somehow to this time constant of the auditory system.

Fortunately, Professor Li Xu from Ohio University was able to provide the large collection of speech probes from a sufficient number of Chinese speakers that was necessary to answer this question. The goal of Xu's research is to understand the mechanisms of hearing and speech perception under electrical stimulation (Xu and Pfingst, 2008) and thus to find ways to improve speech and music perception in patients with cochlear implants (see Section 4.1). Unfortunately, the current technology cannot reliably provide the subtle pitch contours that convey the meaning of words in tonal languages, such as Mandarin (Zhou *et al.*, 2013).

There are only four different so-called 'tones' in Mandarin (T1, T2, T3 and T4). Their pitch contours, which in all four tones include segments of more or less constant pitches, are illustrated in a simplified scheme in Fig. 5.6. While T1 has a nearly constant pitch, T2 is mostly falling, T3 is first falling and then rising and T4 is mostly falling. If they are pronounced as [ma:], T1 means 'mother', T2 'hemp', T3 means 'horse' and T4 'to grumble'.

Diana Deutsch has already demonstrated that the variation of pitch between repetitions of the same tone by the same speaker may be quite small, that is, in the order of a semi-tone (about 6%) or smaller, even if produced on different days (Deutsch *et al.*, 2006). An example for the temporal course of T1 revealing the constancy and convergence to a certain pitch is given for two female speakers in Fig. 5.7. In these cases the pitches converge quite consistently to certain integer multiples (10× and 11×) of 0.4 ms. On the other hand, single subjects are not totally fixed to a particular pitch of each of their tones and the inter-individual variability within groups of children, females and males extends over about an octave. This is also obvious in conscientious pitch measurements provided by Li Xu and colleagues. Based on their extensive material I evaluated 11 repetitions of the four tones of the Mandarin dialect uttered by 56 female and 35 male adult Chinese-Americans (11 repetitions) and 40 repetitions uttered by 180 Chinese children (Fig. 5.8). For the adult subjects a segment of each of their 11 repetitions of the T1 was assumed to have a constant pitch when its standard deviation was less than 1% (<5% for T2–T4). In contrast, the high number of children allowed the evaluation of just a single average pitch value for each subject and tone.

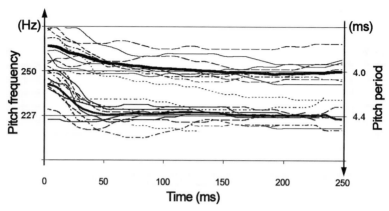

Fig. 5.7   The curves represent 11 repetitions of tone 1 by two Chinese speakers. On average (bold lines) their Chinese pitch periods converge to certain integer (10, 11) multiples of 0.4 ms.

The resulting distributions of dominant pitch periods of the tones show that – as one would expect – children, women and men have different but overlapping ranges of voice pitches, with women about one octave higher than men. In addition, the distributions for the constant pitch periods of the four tones have maxima that correspond approximately to integer multiples of 0.4 ms. Moreover, they are arranged in more or less regular intervals along the axes of pitch periods that correspond to about 0.4 ms for the group of children. For the female and the male group the first two intervals (T4–T1, T1–T2) are 0.8 ms and 1.2 ms, respectively, while the third intervals (T2–T3) are 0.4 ms and 0.8 ms, respectively. Note that for the male group this holds only for the side peak of the T3 distribution at 10 ms, while its major peak coincides with the maximum of the distribution for T2 at 9.2 ms. Note also that several curves have additional side peaks that are also close to certain multiples of 0.4 ms. Strangely enough, for the groups of children and females the distribution of pitches of T1, which has the longest constant pitch segments with the smallest scatter, show the largest deviation from the suggested scheme. This is probably due to the fact that two adjacent integer multiples of 0.4 ms are both likely candidates for individual pitch preference, like in the examples shown for 4.0 and 4.4 ms in Fig. 5.7.

In summary, although the distributions of constant pitch ranges for all subject groups are quite broad and overlapping, their relation to the auditory time constant is evident. This is the case in spite of the fact that even single subjects may make use of different pitches. It seems that for the production of their tones subjects use the multiples of 0.4 ms as benchmarks, but also have the option for additional pitch variations.

5.5   The mystery of flute tuning

At the beginning of the last century the prestigious fathers of music-ethnology, Carl Stumpf (see Fig. 12.1) and Erich von Hornbostel, made a very strange discovery: they found that the fundamental pitch of various musical instruments, such as flutes collected from the South Seas and gamelan instruments from Indonesia, were often tuned with

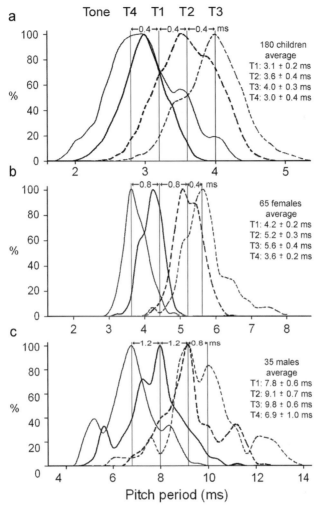

Fig. 5.8   Each of the four normalized distributions in **(a)**, **(b)** and **(c)** is based on 40 **(a)** or 10 **(b,c)** repetitions of one of the four 'tones' (1–4) of the Mandarin dialect by Chinese-Americans. As one would expect, children, women and men have different, but overlapping ranges of voice pitches. In addition, the pitch histograms are arranged in more or less regular distances along the pitch axes that are equivalent for each group. (Note that the average values given differ somewhat from the maxima of the curves.) **(a)** For children (180 subjects), the maxima of the four histograms may be related to the four vertical lines that designate subsequent integer multiples of 0.4 ms (n = 7, 8, 9, 10). **(b)** For the female group (65 subjects), the maxima of the histograms may be related to the four vertical lines, that again designate integer multiples of 0.4 ms (n = 9, 11, 13, 14) with two intervals of 0.8 and one of 0.4 ms. **(c)** For the male group (35 subjects), the resulting maxima are located at 17, 20 and 23 times 0.4 ms with intervals of 1.2 ms. All curves have side peaks close to other multiples of 0.4 ms; this is most obvious in the male group. For example, the curve for tone 3 has a strong side peak close to 25 · 0.4 ms.

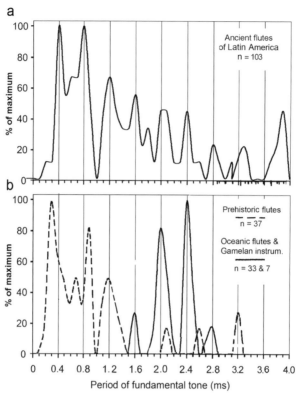

Fig. 5.9   The distribution of fundamental tones of 87 ancient flutes from South America and Mexico, some of them probably more than 2000 years old. The fundamental tones of 46 flutes were determined acoustically (courtesy of Ulrich Hoffmann, Gallery Old-America, Stuttgart, Germany), and 41 fundamental tones were computed from geometric measurements (Ellen Hickmann, 2007). The preference for tunings at fundamental periods that are integer multiples of 0.4 ms is highly significant (Gauss-test, 0.40 ± 0.01, $p < 0.1\%$). **(a)** Carl Stumpf found that flutes from the South Seas, South America (33) and gamelan instruments from Indonesia (7) were often tuned to the same pitch (Stumpf, 1939). As shown, they cluster around integer multiples of 0.4 ms ($n = 4$–7; Gauss-test: 0.40 ms ± 0.01 ms, $p < 0.1\%$). **(b)** Although less significant, the same is true for 37 prehistoric flutes, according to geometric measures published by Clodoré-Tissot (2009) and others ($n = 1$–8; Gauss-test: 0.4 ms ± 0.1 ms, $p < 5\%$).

surprising precision to the same tones (Hornbostel, 1928; Kunst, 1948). The same was true for panpipes from Bolivia, Peru and the Solomon Islands. In his book about epistemology Carl Stumpf mentioned these mysterious findings and still found it quite hard to explain them (Stumpf, 1940). His final conclusion was that of a 'common origin', especially since a 'general necessity, especially of the human hearing system that would constrain people of distant parts of the world to tune their instruments to the same pitches was not apparent' (translations from Stumpf, 1939).

Obviously, Carl Stumpf had thought of an auditory property as the right explanation for the universal tuning phenomenon. Nevertheless, he preferred the quite unlikely assumption of unknown worldwide intercultural contacts as a basis of absolute and identical tuning. After the foregoing we may guess that his rejected hypothesis was the correct one. As a matter of fact, the builders of the flutes (33) and gamelan instruments (7) collected and measured by von Hornbostel and Stumpf had used preferentially multiples (4–7) of 0.4 ms as their tuning benchmarks. This fact is illustrated by the continuous line in Fig. 5.9b. In addition, the broken line shows the distribution of fundamental pitches of a number of prehistoric flutes determined from geometric measures (length and inner diameter) published by Clodoré-Tissot (2009) and others. Amazingly, the fundamental tones of even these extremely old instruments (more than 2000 years) cluster significantly around certain integer (1–8) multiples of 0.4 ms.

Finally, as shown in Fig. 5.9a, the same tone preferences may also be found in the distribution of fundamental tones of 103 ancient flutes from South America and Mexico that I found in the Gallery Old-America, in Stuttgart, Germany and in a corresponding catalogue (Hickmann, 2007). The fundamental pitches of about half of these up to 2000-year-old flutes were determined acoustically, while those of the others were computed from their geometric measures. Yet again, the preference for tunings to fundamental periods that are integer multiples of 0.4 ms is quite evident and even highly significant.

A century after Carl Stumpf's and Erich von Hornbostel's amazing discovery it still remains a mystery why so many musical instruments from all over the world in historic and even prehistoric times are tuned to certain well-defined pitches. Obviously, flute makers must have had not only the desire but also the capacity to tune their instruments in this way. Therefore, a necessary conclusion seems to be that they had some kind of absolute pitch, but naturally not tuned to our diatonic scale with the chamber tone of 440 Hz. Instead they must have had a natural intrinsic reference, the auditory time constant of 0.4 ms.

5.6   The auditory time constant in bird calls

A few years ago a Korean composer won a prize for his innovative compositions at the Holiday Courses for New Music in Darmstadt, Germany. To the amazement of the audience he started his acceptance speech with the confession that he was quite unsure about the quality of his own music. His doubts were due to the observation that his dog would crawl under the sofa whenever he played one of his own compositions, reappearing only after he changed to classical music. Indeed, animals, especially dogs, can be quite picky about sound and music. There were also reports that certain dogs may even have absolute pitch. In addition, wolves and rats are suspected to use absolute pitch information to identify members of their own pack (Levitin and Rogers, 2005).

Perhaps better known is the capability of certain birds, like starlings, to make use of absolute pitch references (Hulse and Cynx, 1985). Therefore, it may not come as a surprise that the auditory benchmark of 0.4 ms may also be uncovered in bird vocalizations. By using various internet sources (e.g. eulenwelt.de, soundbible.com) I found enough examples of vocalizations of different species of cuckoos and owls to come up with reasonable statistics. Fig. 5.10 shows some selected vocalizations as sonagrams and oscillograms. The

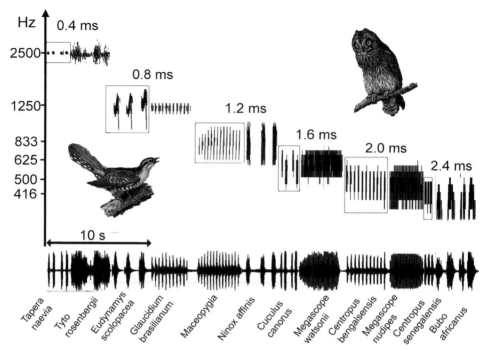

Fig. 5.10   Sonagrams of the vocalizations framed of different species of owls and cuckoos (cuckoo sonagrams
are framed) are quite variable and cover a frequency range from about 200 Hz to about 4000 Hz
(species names are below the oscillograms at the bottom). The selected vocalizations suggest that
there may exist a preference for dominant frequencies with periods in multiples of 0.4 ms.

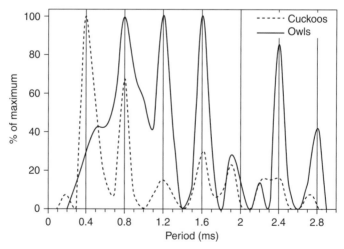

Fig. 5.11   Spectral preferences of vocalizations of different species of cuckoos and owls. The
distributions of the spectral maxima of vocalizations from 128 birds (72 owls and 56 cuckoos)
show preferences for signal periods that are integer multiples of 0.4 ms (n = 1–7; Gauss-test,
0.40 ms ± 0.05 ms, $p < 0.1\%$ for cuckoos and $p < 1\%$ for owls).

frequency range covered by different species extends over a wide range from about 200 Hz to about 4000 Hz, with significant numbers of these birds keeping their voice periods close to integer multiples of 0.4 ms. This becomes quite obvious from the distributions of the spectral maxima of a reasonable number (128) of these bird calls (Fig. 5.11). This simple measure works fine in this case, since birds often produce relatively long, sometimes even pure tones, with modulations restricted to comparatively small frequency ranges (see Fig. 5.10). Obviously, the spectral maxima of the evaluated bird calls cluster again significantly around integer multiples (1–7) of 0.4 ms. Therefore, at least some species of birds must have and make use of the same auditory benchmark as humans. Indeed, in Chapter 8 it will be shown that the underlying temporal intervals in the auditory system can be demonstrated in neurophysiological experiments in various animals, including birds. Probably they are the result of intrinsic oscillations in the first processing centre of the auditory system, the cochlear nucleus.

Finally, it remains an open question which other species of birds (and perhaps also of mammals) may have the same frequency preferences as cuckoos and owls. By means of standard computer equipment and the facility of the internet, it should be easy for the experienced reader to find more evidence.

6   Pathways of hearing

6.1   From the cochlea to the cortex

Acoustic signals transferred from the outer to the inner ear elicit neural signals in the cochlea that travel in the form of nerve impulses along the auditory pathways. They follow ascending fibre tracts from the brainstem to the midbrain and from there through the thalamus to the cerebral cortex (Fig. 6.1). Each of these fibre tracts contains many thousands of nerve fibres (axons) that connect the nerve cells of a series of auditory processing centres (nuclei).

The auditory nerve connects the cochlea with the entrance station to the central auditory system, the cochlear nucleus (CN). From here, acoustic information travels to the inferior colliculus via both direct and indirect routes. This midbrain nucleus is a major processing centre for all auditory information on its way to the cortex. It receives input from the CN on both sides, from the nuclei of the lateral lemniscus and also from the superior olivary complex (containing binaural information). As we will see (Chapters 8–11), the inferior colliculus also plays a central role in periodicity processing and therefore also in this book.

The next level of the auditory pathway is the medial geniculate body, located in the thalamus. This nucleus is often considered as the gateway to the auditory cortex that forms part of the cortical temporal lobe. Here fundamental acoustic features like timbre, pitch, loudness and localization, which have already been analysed in the lower processing centres, are processed further. Finally, fibres of descending (efferent) pathways course downwards from the cortex and other auditory areas to influence the lower processing centres. They provide a negative feedback, or inhibitory control, which influences the sensitivity and selectivity of these nuclei.

6.2   The ear

6.2.1   The receiving system

Our ear consists of three main parts: the outer, middle and the inner ear (Fig. 6.2). The pinna and ear canal of the outer ear collect sound waves and guide them to the eardrum (*tympanic membrane*). The acoustic waves give rise to vibrations of this membrane and the attached chain of tiny ear bones in the middle ear. They are the smallest bones in our body and

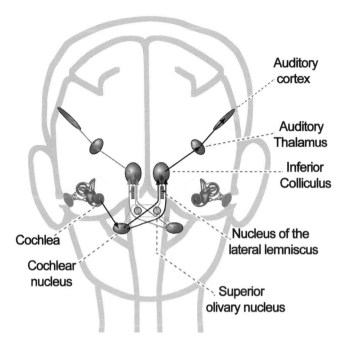

Fig. 6.1   A simplified scheme of the way acoustic information is transmitted from the outer ear to the auditory cortex. Not shown are the massive back projections from most of the nuclei, especially from the cortex to the thalamus.

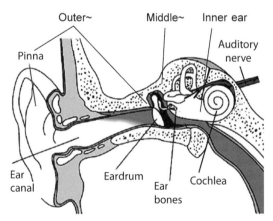

Fig. 6.2   Acoustic waves collected by the pinna pass through the external ear canal, and give rise to vibrations on the eardrum and the attached tiny bones of the middle ear: the hammer, anvil and stirrup. This chain of bones transfers the sound signals to the cochlea in the inner ear. Receptor cells in the cochlea transpose the acoustic information into a neural ('spike') code which is then sent to the brain via the auditory nerve (modified from Pickles, 1988).

basically act as a system of mechanical levers. Because of their characteristic shapes, and irrespective of their minuscule size, they have been named the hammer, anvil and stirrup (in Latin: malleus, incus and stapes).

The stirrup is the last bone in this chain; its footplate contacts the fluid-filled cavities of the helically shaped cochlea in the inner ear through a small opening in the bone called the oval window. As the ear bones have a lever function and, moreover, the area of the oval window is much smaller than that of the eardrum, the pressure is 22 times higher at the oval window than at the eardrum. On the other hand, the displacement of the vibration is reduced, so that the whole transformation leads to a match of the acoustic impedances (ratio of sound pressure to the velocity of molecules of an acoustic medium) of the environmental air and the liquid of the inner ear. Otherwise, most of the sound energy would be reflected from the cochlear fluid, which is heavy (dense) and incompressible in comparison to the air.

6.2.2   The cochlea

The cochlea is the site where all the information contained within a sound is converted into neural activity. The mechanical vibrations of the eardrum and middle ear are first converted into hydraulic pressure waves and then, by receptor cells, into action potentials (spikes, see Box 6.1).

When the footplate of the stapes vibrates in response to sound, the oval window is moved inwards and pressure waves are induced in two fluid-filled compartments or

---

BOX 6.1 The nerve cell

The elementary module of all nervous systems is the nerve cell or neuron. Usually, neurons have a cell body from which two types of appendices, the dendrites and one axon, extend. A neuron may have thousands of synaptic inputs at its dendrites or cell body, but it has always only one output, the axon, that may, however, split to form multiple branches (collaterals). Neurons communicate with each other by sending a standardized electrical signal, the action potential ('spike') along their axons.

Because of their intra- and extracellular ionic concentrations, all cells have a negative membrane potential (resting potential) of about −60 mV. Their sodium channels open after a synaptic activation; positive sodium ions pour in and increase (depolarize) the membrane potential of the cells. Provided the depolarization is too strong to be compensated by the immediate efflux of positively charged potassium ions, voltage-sensitive sodium channels will open; more sodium ions pour in and the depolarization increases. Once the membrane potential reaches a certain threshold (about −30 mV) the number of open sodium channels snowballs and within less than a millisecond the potential changes by about 90 mV, from −60 to +30 mV. The whole process is known as the 'Hodgkin–Huxley cycle'. When the sodium channels close again an increased efflux from the intracellular potassium pool repolarizes the cell, but it takes a few milliseconds (refractory period) until the resting potential is reached and the cell is ready to 'spike' again.

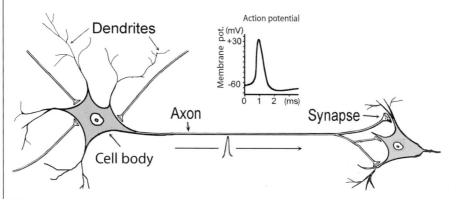

Fig. 6.1.1

The excitation of the cell membrane spreads along the nerve fibre. The speed of the 'spike' (1–100 m/s) depends on the diameter of the fibre, but even more so on its insulation (myelinization). After reaching the synapses at the ends of the axon, transmitter molecules are released from their storage sites (vesicles) and open ion channels at the membrane of the next cell. There are excitatory synapses with transmitters which open sodium channels (e.g. glutamate) and inhibitory synapses with transmitters (e.g. GABA or glycine) which open potassium or chloride channels. If the receiving cell receives more excitatory than inhibitory input it will respond with an action potential (see above).

canals, the *scala vestibuli* and *scala tympani* (Fig. 6.3). These canals are joined through a small opening at the apex of the spiral. At the base of the scala tympani is another opening, the round window, covered by a membrane which moves outwards when the oval window is pushed inwards – this compensates for the pressure changes in the almost incompressible fluid (*perilymph*) in the two scalae.

The whole system is so minute that it takes only a fraction of a millilitre of perilymph to fill the canals. The scalae vestibuli and tympani are separated by a third duct, the cochlear duct or *scala media*, which contains fluid with a somewhat different ionic composition (*endolymph*). The endolymph of this compartment is separated from the perilymph of the scala vestibuli by a thin membrane, Reissner's membrane, and from the scala tympani by the *basilar membrane*.

6.2.3   The travelling wave

As we have seen in Chapter 3, in the mid nineteenth century Hermann von Helmholtz put forward his resonance theory in which he hypothesized that the cochlea functions like a Fourier analyser; its main task was to represent the spectrum of acoustic signals. In 1928 Georg von Békésy, a telecommunications engineer at the Hungarian Post Office

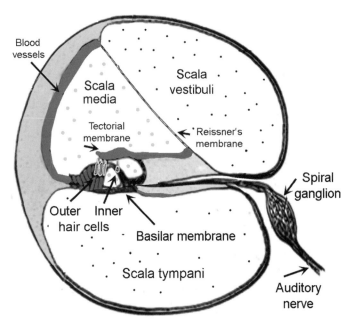

Fig 6.3   The helically coiled cochlea has three fluid-filled compartments or canals, the scala vestibuli, the scala media and the scala tympani. On top of the basilar membrane sits the organ of Corti. Its three rows of outer and one row of inner hair cells are capped by the tectorial membrane.

in Budapest, introduced a new and more accurate theory of basilar membrane function, which revolutionized our understanding of how the cochlea processes sound. More than 30 years later, in 1961, von Békésy received the Nobel Prize in Physiology, the only auditory scientist as yet to have been given this honour.

In a series of amazingly elegant experiments using mechanical models of the cochlea, von Békésy filled metal tubes with water and stretched a membrane along the length of the tube. He observed that vibrations elicited waves sweeping along the membrane – he called these 'travelling waves' (Fig. 6.4). By using flakes of silver as a marker and strobe photography he was able to actually see such waves on the basilar membranes of ears dissected from human cadavers and animals, including an elephant from the zoo in Budapest.

In our ear, the basilar membrane runs almost the whole length of the cochlea (~36 mm), but both its stiffness and its width differ along its length (Fig. 6.4). Contrary to what one might expect from the outer shape of the cochlea, at its base (i.e. at the oval window) the basilar membrane is narrow, only about 0.1 mm wide, but at the apex it has broadened to a width of 0.5 mm (Pickles, 1988). In addition, the stiffness of the membrane decreases by a factor of about 10 000 from the base to the apex. As a result of these mechanical properties, a pure tone elicits a wave in the cochlea which moves along the membrane. It is the frequency of the tone that determines the place on the basilar membrane at which the travelling wave reaches its maximum. After this point, the wave is decelerated and collapses rapidly because of frictional forces.

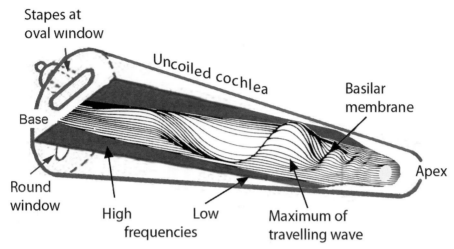

Stapes at
oval window

Uncoiled cochlea

Basilar
membrane

Base

Round
window

High

Low

frequencies

Maximum of
travelling wave

Apex

Fig. 6.4   This schematic diagram shows the uncoiled cochlea (proportions are not accurate). The stirrup
transfers acoustic vibrations to the cochlea through the oval window. A pure tone elicits a
simple wave that travels along the basilar membrane. If the frequency changes from
high to low, the wave maximum shifts from locations near the base to locations near the apex
(modified from Tonndorf, 1960).

So for each input frequency there is a certain place on our basilar membrane which will
respond maximally and, as a consequence, we are able to discriminate between different
frequencies. Just as von Helmholtz had originally postulated, von Békésy proved that
high-frequency tones excite sensory cells near the base of the cochlea and lower frequencies excite cells towards the apex. This systematic representation of frequency in the
cochlea is nowadays known as the tonotopic organization (sometimes more correctly
named 'cochleotopy'). We now know that the cochlear analysis results in a tonotopic
representation of frequency in all auditory processing centres up to the cortex (see below).

Just as for many other aspects of auditory processing, investigations of travelling
wave mechanisms focused on the consequences of pure tone stimulation. However, the
main task of the cochlea is actually the processing of complex sounds, like those in
animal and human communication. As we know from the previous chapters, these are
often harmonic sounds with many frequency components (harmonics). Consequently,
decomposition of such signals must be a major task of cochlear sound analysis. In
essence, in this analysis frequency components are mapped to frequency-specific places
of maximal response along the basilar membrane and the neuronal response of the
receptor cells (hair cells, see Box 6.2) located at these places codes their amplitudes.

The decomposition of harmonic sounds in the cochlea is incomplete, because only the
three to four lowest harmonics are well resolved and give rise to separated maxima of the
travelling wave. As frequencies are mapped on a logarithmic scale along the basilar
membrane, the higher harmonics increasingly overlap and remain partly or even completely unresolved.

Their vibrations sum up and create beating patterns that vary in complexity. But two
interfering vibrations always beat with a frequency which is equal to their difference

BOX 6.2 The organ of Corti

The organ of Corti is localized on top of the basilar membrane and contains hair cells, supporting cells (not shown) and the endings of the auditory nerve. It is capped by the tectorial membrane (not shown). Altogether about 15 000 hair cells are arranged along the length of the basilar membrane in an orderly fashion in four rows, one 'inner' row and three 'outer' rows.

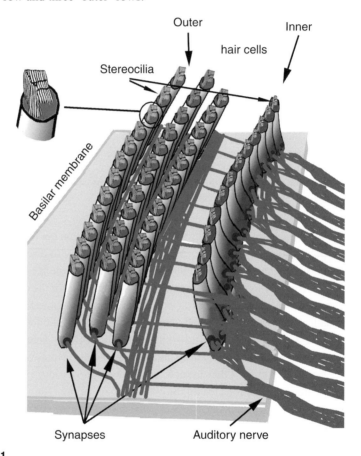

Fig. 6.2.1

Each inner hair cell has 20–50 tiny processes or stereocilia that protrude in a nice arrangement like organ pipes from the top of each cell. The stereocilia are arranged in several rows, interconnected with their neighbours by 'tip links'. The relative movements of the basilar, the tectorial membrane and of the surrounding fluid deflect the stereocilia in the rhythm of the stimulating frequency.

The bending of the stereocilia stretches their tip links and this causes their ion channels to open in the rhythm of their oscillations. Since the fluid surrounding the hair cells contains a high concentration of positively charged ions, mainly potassium and calcium, these ions follow the electrical gradient and flow inwards when the corresponding ion channels open. The resulting depolarization of the cell is called a receptor potential. It causes the hair cells to release the transmitter glutamate into the attached terminals of the auditory nerve at the cell base.

The main receptors of our hearing system are the *inner hair cells*; they transfer the acoustic information into a neural code. Each of these cells is contacted by about 20 nerve fibres. In contrast, the main function of the *outer hair cells* is to amplify weak acoustic vibrations by actively changing their length in the rhythm of the impinging sound wave. This amplification is controlled by the innervation of the outer hair cells originating in the brainstem. The corresponding nerve fibres run in a spiral direction along the basilar membrane and contact many outer hair cells.

frequency. As we know from Chapters 2 and 3, all frequencies of a harmonic sound are integer multiples of its fundamental frequency. Therefore, the beating pattern on many places along the basilar membrane will have a frequency that is equal to the frequency of the fundamental component. It is important to keep in mind that this is a purely temporal phenomenon and that there is no change in the spectral composition, at least as long as the sound intensity is not too high and distortions are negligible. In this book I emphasize this temporal aspect of wave mechanics by using the term 'periodicity' over the corresponding term 'frequency'.

6.2.4   The organ of Corti

The most important part of the cochlea is the delicate and highly sensitive *organ of Corti*, named after its discoverer Alfonso Corti (1822–1876). The organ of Corti consists of thousands of sensory receptor cells that are arranged in four rows along the basilar membrane (see Box 6.2). These cells have a tuft of hair-like stereocilia that protrudes from their top and are therefore also known as hair cells. Their function is to transform acoustic into neural information.

In response to the travelling waves, the stereocilia of the hair cells bend, similar to sheaves of wheat bending in the wind. An upward movement of the basilar membrane stretches the links that interconnect the stereocilia and opens their ion channels. The resulting inward current depolarizes the membrane potential of the hair cells, while a downward movement of the membrane has the opposite effect (Fig. 6.5). As a consequence, most spikes are generated during the upward movement in the nerve fibres connected to the hair cells, followed by a pause or reduction of the firing.

A sound signal with a higher amplitude will result in a higher amplitude of the travelling wave and therefore also in stronger bending of the stereocilia. This opens more channels, increases the ion currents and the depolarization, and finally activates the nerve fibres.

Moreover, when the amplitude of the signal changes periodically, the average response is modulated accordingly and therefore reflects not only the amplitude but also the periodicity of the envelope, as well as of the temporal fine structure of the signal (Fig. 6.5). This mechanism is effective in the frequency range below about 5 kHz, the upper limit of phase coupling or synchronization.

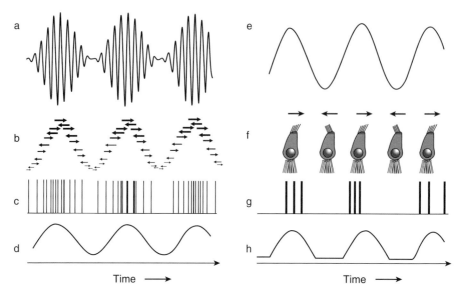

Fig. 6.5   (a) A section of an AM signal. (b) The arrows indicate the amplitude, the time course and the
direction of movement of the cilia of a hair cell due to the signal. (c) Action potentials (here
simplified as lines) are elicited when the signal amplitude is high. (d) The average response
reflects the periodicity of the envelope. (e) Enlargement, showing only the three waves in the box
(a). (f) The cilia are bending with the same period as the sound, thereby opening and closing
ion channels. (g) Action potentials are elicited when the cilia are bent in the right direction.
(h) The response reflects also the temporal fine structure of the signal.

6.2.5   The cochlear amplifier

The vast range of sound intensities that we can hear is truly remarkable. The difference
in intensity, or loudness, between sounds that are barely perceptible (such as the rustling
of a mouse) and those on the threshold of causing pain (such as the roar of a jet plane)
depends on the frequency of the sound, but can be up to a trillion-fold (a factor of one
million million). The extreme sensitivity of our ear cannot be explained by the passive
mechanism of the travelling wave alone. In the absence of any clear evidence, scientists
speculated for decades that there must be additional mechanisms present in the inner ear
that could explain both the high sensitivity and the narrow tuning of fibres in the auditory
nerve. What was needed was some sort of cochlear amplifier that was capable of actively
increasing the intensity of weak sound signals by a factor of about 10 000, or 40 dB (for
an explanation of the decibel scale, see Box 6.3). It is only some 30 years ago that Jim
Hudspeth finally found this amplifier in the three rows of outer hair cells (see Box 6.2).

Until Hudspeth's amazing discovery, the function of the approximately 12 000 outer
hair cells was a complete mystery, since nearly all (95%) of the nerve fibres that transmit
information to the brain contact only the ~3500 inner hair cells. The depolarization of the
outer hair cells drives them to actively contract in the rhythm of the stimulating
frequency. The rapid change in length is quite comparable to a muscle contraction and
requires energy; this is provided by the densely packed blood vessels at the outer wall of
the inner ear (see Fig. 6.3).

BOX 6.3 The Bel scale

Since we perceive sound logarithmically over a large range of intensity, it is measured on a logarithmic scale, the Bel scale (B). A certain B value x tells how much louder the sound intensity I (measured in Watt/m²) is than a reference I_0. If the reference I_0 (p_0) is the human hearing threshold at 1 kHz, the scale is labelled as SPL (sound pressure level).

For practical reasons, one multiplies the logarithm by 10 and uses dB (= B/10) instead of B. The 10 turns into 20 when intensity is replaced by sound pressure (measured in Newton m^{-2}), because intensity is proportional to the square of pressure:

$$X \, dB \, SPL = 10\log\left(\tfrac{I}{I_0}\right) = 10\log\left(\tfrac{p^2}{p_0^2}\right) = 20\log\left(\tfrac{p}{p_0}\right).$$

Since our hearing threshold is at about 0 dB SPL and our pain threshold is reached at about 120 dB SPL, our dynamic range of hearing corresponds to a ratio of sound intensities of 10^{12} (one trillion). We whisper at about 20, talk at 65 and shout at 80 dB SPL.

An increase of 20 dB means the pressure has increased by a factor of 10 and the corresponding intensity by a factor of 100. Three dB corresponds to a doubling of intensity and 6 dB to a doubling of sound pressure.

The active movements of the outer hair cells result in a stronger movement of the basilar membrane and therefore in stronger responses of the adjacent inner hair cells. As the outer hair cells resonate at their particular frequencies, both the amplitude of the travelling wave and the frequency tuning are enhanced in a specific region of the cochlea (Hudspeth, 1997). Finally, the minority of nerve fibres (about 5%) that make multiple contacts with the outer hair cells play a crucial role in controlling their responses and thus in adapting the sensitivity of hearing.

6.3   The auditory nerve

6.3.1   Spectral coding

The cell bodies of auditory nerve fibres (ganglion cells) are located in the spiral ganglion in the centre of the cochlea (see Fig. 6.3). Electrophysiological recordings from the auditory nerve show that the cochlea functions as a filter bank, with the auditory nerve fibres serving as output channels that transfer spectral and temporal information from the hair cells to nerve cells in the brainstem. If fibres receive their input from different locations (hair cells) on the basilar membrane they will respond best to different frequencies (characteristic frequencies = CF) and their discharge rate will depend on the amplitude of these frequencies (Fig. 6.6). The distribution of activity in the auditory nerve thus forms an image of the sound spectrum of a signal.

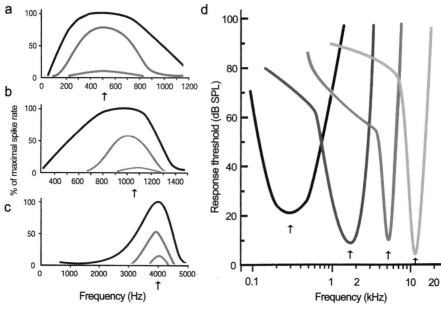

Fig. 6.6   **(a)–(c)** Schemes of three typical responses of auditory nerve fibres (as measured in detail, e.g. in the squirrel monkey by Rose *et al.*, 1971). The curves indicate responses at different intensities (near threshold: light grey; medium intensity: medium grey; high intensity: black); in order to elicit a response at the lowest intensities the stimulus has to have a particular frequency (CF, indicated by arrows). The response curves are much broader at medium and high levels than at the lowest levels, especially below 1 kHz. **(d)** Schemes of four typical tuning curves of auditory nerve fibres (as measured in detail, e.g. in the cat by Javel, 1986). They illustrate the threshold intensity above which the fibres respond to frequency stimuli. The tip of each curve defines the CF of the corresponding nerve fibre (indicated by arrows). The large widths of response and threshold curves show that our high-frequency discrimination (<1%), requires additional temporal analysis in the central auditory system.

We are able to distinguish frequencies which differ by less than 1%; for example, we can distinguish a 1000 Hz tone from a 1003 Hz tone. This would lead us to expect that our auditory nerve fibres are correspondingly tuned. However, although the quality of their tuning increases with frequency, in the range below 5 kHz their filter curves are quite broad in relation to their CFs. This effect is even more obvious at frequencies below 1 kHz and becomes more pronounced with increasing intensity (Fig. 6.6 a, b). It seems that our acute frequency discrimination, below 5 kHz at least, cannot rely on cochlear frequency analysis alone; supplementary temporal coding in the nerve and a corresponding analysis in the central auditory system appears indispensable.

Fortunately, the auditory nerve is not restricted to spectral coding. In addition, its firing patterns contain information about acoustic timing at the two ears, as well as synchronized activity to vibrations, modulations and fluctuations up to about 5 kHz. This temporal information is useful for the discrimination of signals, but it is also required for the binding of the components of complex signals, such as the formants of vowels that are separated by the cochlear filter into different frequency channels. A major task of central auditory processing is to integrate and bind such matching information from different locations (neurons) in the brainstem. Since the temporal modulations or fluctuations of acoustic signals tend to be synchronous over broad frequency ranges, they provide the necessary tags for this binding process.

6.3.2   A limited dynamic range

The capabilities of our hearing system are based on the transfer of acoustic information by many thousands of nerve fibres. In comparison, any single fibre is quite limited in several aspects of coding. One of these aspects is the so-called dynamic range (Fig. 6.7). Information about sound intensity (loudness) is coded in the average firing rate of nerve fibres. The louder the sounds, the more spikes per second are generated in the fibre. However, no matter how loud the sound, the fibre cannot produce more than a few hundred spikes per second, and therefore no single nerve fibre is able to present the full intensity range our hearing system can handle (a small subgroup of fibres which are characterized by high thresholds and low spontaneous activity may play a particular role because they surpass the majority in this respect and may reach a dynamic range of 60–80 dB SPL).

A typical nerve fibre (Fig. 6.7) has a coding range for intensities that is limited to about 30–40 dB (Evans and Palmer, 1980), but with increasing tone intensity our hearing system recruits more and more fibres that either have higher thresholds or are tuned slightly different and therefore need higher sound amplitudes to be activated.

Just exactly how such information arising from different fibres is integrated by the central hearing system is not quite clear, but neurons have been found in central processing centres which indeed have higher dynamic ranges. The limitation of the dynamic range is a drawback for intensity coding, but it is also a necessary prerequisite for temporal processing mechanisms (Chapters 7–9).

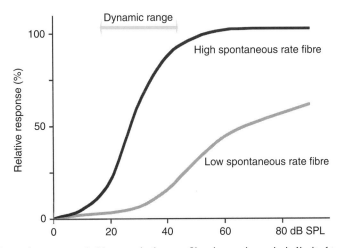

Fig. 6.7   The intensity range coded by a typical nerve fibre in a guinea pig is limited to about 30–40 dB (modified after Winter *et al.*, 1990).

6.3.3   Temporal coding

The vibrations of the hair cells follow the peaks and valleys of the acoustic waves precisely, even up to the very highest audible frequencies (see Fig. 6.5). As a consequence, the membrane potentials of the hair cells are also synchronized, even at high frequencies (Fig. 6.8). This is true in spite of a rectifying effect due to the fact that the ion channels close in one direction of their oscillating movements (see Fig. 6.5h).

   The duration of a single spike is about 1 ms and, in addition, each spike is followed by a refractory period which may last for a few milliseconds (see Box 6.1). As a consequence the maximal spike rate even of a fast neuron is limited to frequencies well below 1 kHz. How, then, can frequencies up to 5 kHz be temporally coded in the nerve?

   Interestingly, William Rutherford was forced to address this problem when he postulated, in the nineteenth century, that the ear functions like the newly invented telephone, in spite of the fact that the firing rates observed in animal nerves were only in the order of several hundred Hertz (see Section 4.1). More than half a century later, in 1949, Ernest Glen Wever proposed a possible solution, putting forward his famous principle of frequency coding, known now as Wever's *volley principle* (Fig. 6.9; Wever, 1949).

   As is often the case with great ideas, the volley principle is quite simple. As phase coding follows statistical rules, two adjacent fibres have a probability of firing at different cycles of an acoustic signal. Although no single nerve fibre is able to code all cycles of a high-frequency sound in a one-to-one relationship, the combined firing of a

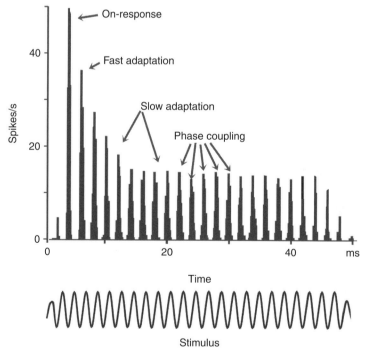

Fig. 6.8   A typical auditory nerve fibre synchronizes in response to its CF of 500 Hz (example from the chinchilla, 200 repetitions of a tone, 50 ms duration, 65 dB SPL).

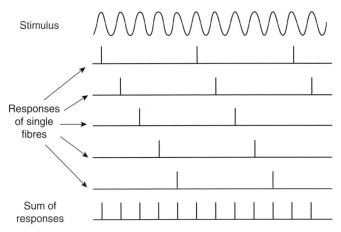

Stimulus

Responses
of single
fibres

Sum of
responses

Fig. 6.9   According to *Wever's volley principle*, temporal coding may extend to frequencies as high
as 5 kHz by utilizing parallel coding in several adjacent nerve fibres (it is not necessary for the
principle that the spike intervals are all the same).

sufficient number of fibres, each synchronized to a different cycle, may code temporal
information of frequencies up to about 5 kHz.

Thus, according to the volley principle, temporal information can be transferred via
the auditory nerve up to frequencies of about 5 kHz, suggesting that the neuronal
mechanisms underlying the perception of pitch involve temporal processing
(Greenberg, 1988). Accordingly, the upper limit of musical pitch perception, defined
by the ability to recognize musical intervals, is also at about 5 kHz (Semal and Demany,
1990).

However, although the temporal information carried by the volleys of spikes in a
group of fibres may be useful for the analysis of frequency information in the brain,
major questions are still waiting to be answered: How is this information decoded in the
subsequent brain centres? Which of their neurons are able to make use of this information? How do they do this? Probable answers are presented in Chapter 9.

6.4   Cochlear nucleus

6.4.1   Functional organization

Fibres of the auditory nerve terminate in the first auditory processing centre in the
brainstem, the cochlear nucleus (CN). This nucleus is very similar in all mammals,
including man, and receives its information about acoustic signals from the auditory
nerve fibres. Its task is to transform and distribute information to several parallel neural
pathways in a way which allows subsequent centres to derive the relevant parameters of
sounds.

The CN is divided into three subnuclei: the anterior ventral cochlear nucleus
(AVCN), the posterior ventral cochlear nucleus (PVCN) and the dorsal cochlear nucleus

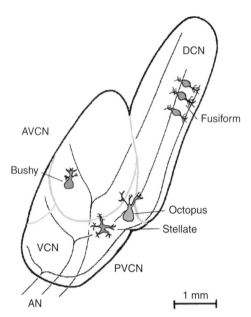

Fig. 6.10   The dorsal (DCN) and ventral (VCN) cochlear nucleus, the latter subdivided into an anterior (AVCN) and posterior (PVCN) part, are shown together with the four major neuron types (further subdivisions and subclasses of cells are ignored). All four depicted neuron types are projection neurons. For example, stellate and fusiform cells project directly to the inferior colliculus and octopus cells to the ventral nucleus of the lateral lemniscus (modified from Moore and Osen, 1979).

(DCN) (Fig. 6.10). After reaching the CN, the auditory nerve fibres bifurcate into a dorsal and a ventral branch, with the result that identical auditory information is carried into these different regions. Thorough investigations in many animals showed that the tonotopic map – arising in the cochlea – is systematically represented in all three subnuclei of the CN. The four major neuron types of the CN (Fig. 6.10) give rise to widespread projections to nuclei throughout the brainstem (Cant and Benson, 2003).

Many studies have used an anatomical technique, known as intracellular horseradish peroxidase labelling, to correlate morphological cell types with physiological response patterns (e.g. Kavanagh *et al.*, 1979; Rhode *et al.*, 1983a, 1983b; Rouiller and Ryugo, 1984; Oertel *et al.*, 1988). Therefore it is now well known that, for example, bushy cells project to the olivary nuclei and provide highly precise directional information for binaural processing. Importantly for the temporal analysis of pitch (Chapter 9), a subgroup of stellate cells (T-stellate cells) project to the auditory midbrain (inferior colliculus) on the opposite side of the brain (Osen, 1969). It is also essential for periodicity processing that octopus cells project to the ventral part of the nucleus of the lateral lemniscus (see Chapter 11), a pathway present in all mammals and especially prominent in humans (Adams, 1997).

The response characteristics of different cell types arise partly from their different morphologies and membrane properties, and partly from the intricate connections

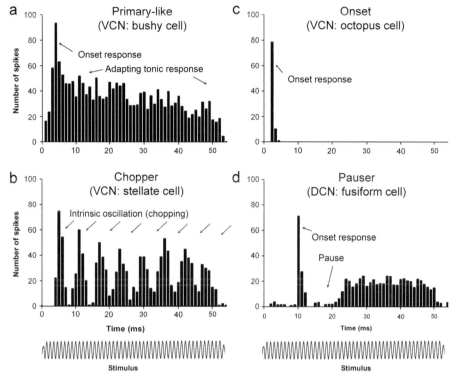

Fig. 6.11   Schemes of the four major response types in the CN as have been observed in various animals and also humans (e.g. Pfeiffer, 1966). The responses may be elicited by stimulation with a pure tone at the CFs of the neurons. The stimulus waveform at the bottom is out of scale to indicate its temporal structure.

among some of the cell types. For the cochlear nucleus four major response types have been described (Fig. 6.11a–d): primary-like (bushy cells), chopper (T-stellate cells), onset (octopus and D-stellate cells) and pauser cells (fusiform and giant cells). All of these response types have been further subdivided into subclasses.

The responses of bushy cells in the anterior VCN are very similar to those of corresponding auditory nerve fibres (Fig. 6.11a). They are characterized by an onset and a tonic response that decreases over time.

T-stellate cells in the posterior VCN are known for their very regular oscillatory (chopper) responses that are unrelated to the stimulus period (Fig. 6.11b). They are either transient or lasting and the oscillation periods in different cells vary from 0.8 to about 10 ms.

Octopus cells in the posterior VCN typically show a strong on-response to pure tones which is very precise (phasic) and has only a short latency (Fig. 6.11c).

Fusiform and giant cells in the posterior VCN also show a strong on-response but with a longer latency followed by a pause of a few milliseconds and a continuous (tonic) response with sometimes extremely regular intervals between individual spikes (Fig. 6.11d).

6.4.2   The ventral part

The auditory nerve fibres make extremely large synaptic contacts (known as *giant synapses* or, more specifically, *endbulbs of Held*) with the spherical bushy cells in the front part of the VCN (Osen, 1988). These contacts are among the largest synapses in the whole central nervous system and may involve major parts of the membrane of the bushy cells. Because of the security of these contacts, there is a high probability that the bushy cell will also generate a spike when a spike invades its giant synapse. As a result, their responses are very similar to those of the auditory nerve (Fig. 6.11a), which is why they are called primary-like (Bourk, 1976). The resulting temporal coding is so precise that it allows our hearing system to measure the difference of arrival times of a sound at our two ears with microsecond precision.

In 1966 R. R. Pfeiffer discovered the intriguing regularly oscillating responses in the CN which he called chopper responses (Fig. 6.11b). He noticed that each chopper cell oscillates in the millisecond range with its own characteristic periodicity, quite independent of the frequency and amplitude of the acoustic signals.

Nowadays, auditory physiologists distinguish three types of choppers (Bourk, 1976; Blackburn and Sachs, 1989). 'Sustained' choppers are characterized by extremely constant spike intervals; with their characteristic intrinsic frequency they may oscillate during the whole presentation time of a stimulus. In contrast, the spike intervals of 'transient' choppers do change to some extent over time. Another group of chopper cells are called 'onset' choppers. They are characterized by prominent onset peaks in addition to their oscillations. The delays introduced by chopper oscillations are suitable to serve as temporal references for the analysis of periodic signals (see Section 9.4.3).

When it comes to onset responses, no cell type surpasses the octopus cells (Fig. 6.11c). They were named by the distinguished Norwegian anatomist Kirsten Osen (1969) because of the resemblance of their dendrites to the tentacles of an octopus (Fig. 6.12). Their long 'arms' enable them to contact many auditory nerve fibres and as a consequence they respond equally well to many frequencies, i.e. they are very broadly tuned (see Fig. 7.5a). They do not 'care' much about frequency and are mostly concerned with timing. To the onset of unmodulated tones above 1.5 kHz they respond with a single, highly synchronized spike and then remain mostly silent (Godfrey *et al.*, 1975; Rhode and Smith, 1986). In contrast, for low frequencies, periodic modulations or clicks they show the strongest synchronous responses of all neurons in the CN (see Figs. 7.5–7.7). One may conclude that these cells must play an important role in the coding and processing of single acoustic events (transients) as well as periodicity information. We will discuss the possibility that octopus cells transfer their precise timing information to chopper neurons in Chapter 9.

6.4.3   The dorsal part

As complex as the organization and functional specialization of the VCN may be, that of the dorsal cochlear nucleus (DCN) is even greater (see Fig. 7.11). Kirsten Osen (1969)

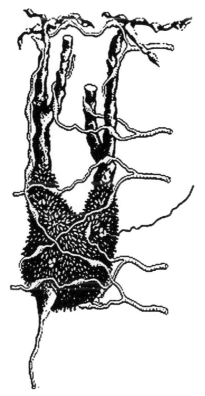

Fig. 6.12 The dendritic arms of the very broadly tuned octopus cells are stretched out to receive input from many nerve fibres (modified from Morest *et al.*, 1973, fig. 2).

named this tiny nucleus 'the cerebellum of the cochlear nucleus'. The reason is that its highly ordered organization mirrors that of the cerebellum (Oertel and Young, 2004), a large structure of our brain that is specialized predominantly for the temporal coordination of precise motor actions.

The response properties of the two output neurons (principal cells) of the DCN – the fusiform and the giant cells – are very similar (Fig. 6.11d). Like the so-called Purkinje cells in the cerebellum, the fusiform cells are arranged in long rows with their dendrites aligned while axons from granule cells, also located in this nucleus, run perpendicular to these dendrites.

The principal cells also get input from the auditory nerve and respond best to a particular tone, their CF, provided the sound level is not more than 20–30 dB above their threshold. At higher levels they are mostly inhibited by pure tones, even by frequencies at their CF (Evans and Nelson, 1973). The principal cells are also called 'pauser cells' because of their remarkable temporal response patterns: their reaction starts with a temporally precise onset, followed, after a short pause, by a slowly increasing weaker response. Quite in contrast to their constrained response to pure tones, they do respond vigorously and with accurate timing to noise (Goldberg and Brownell, 1973; Young and Brownell, 1976). On the other hand, in spite of their strong inhibition in response to pure tones, principal cells may synchronize extremely well to periodic sounds and are therefore able to faithfully code the fluctuations and modulations of acoustic signals (see Chapter 7). Consequently, I will suggest in Chapter 9 that these cells play an important role in temporal coding and periodicity analysis.

6.5   Olivary nuclei

Many cell types in the CN transfer information to higher processing centres, with different cell types having different response properties, different projection pathways and targets. The neuronal structures which receive the binaural temporal and intensity information about sound localization from the bushy cells are the superior olivary nuclei (Fig. 6.1). Because these nuclei receive (direct or indirect) input from both sides of the brain, their neurons are able to compare features of the signal at the two ears.

When our head shadows a signal on one side more than on the other, because the signal source is lateralized, neurons in the lateral superior olive (LSO) are able to compare the different response strength at the two ears. In contrast, neurons in the medical superior olive (MSO) are sensitive to the timing differences in the activation of both ears. They process the difference of the arrival time at the two ears with a precision of 10 µs. As a consequence we are able to localize the direction of a sound within a few degrees. This high binaural accuracy may be considered as an indisputable proof of the power of temporal processing in the auditory system.

In both olivary nuclei, the sensitivities to temporal disparities or intensity differences, respectively, are distributed along the spatial axes of the nuclei and are laid out in topographical maps. Since these maps are the result of neuronal processing or computation, they are also often called 'computational maps'. We will encounter another such computational map for temporal information in the auditory midbrain, in this case for signal periodicities (Chapter 10).

6.6   Lateral lemniscus

Octopus cells do not project directly to the inferior colliculus, but to stellate cells and DCN principal cells; this is an essential aspect of the pitch theory presented in Chapter 9. In addition, they send their axons mostly to the other side of the brain. Their major target is the ventral part of an elongated cell group embedded in the fibres of the lateral lemniscus, located immediately below the inferior colliculus. Besides the ventral nucleus of the lateral lemniscus (VNLL), a dorsal nucleus (DNLL) has been distinguished and in some animals anatomists even recognize three distinct nuclei, all of them sending inhibitory projections to the inferior colliculus (Zhang *et al.*, 1998; Riquelme *et al.*, 2001).

Just like the primary-like cells in the CN, the cells of the VNLL receive their information via giant synapses (Vater *et al.*, 1997). This allows the innervating octopus cells to transmit their (obviously important) information in a temporally highly secure way. Not surprisingly, therefore, many neurons in the VNLL reflect the properties of their octopus cell input and code the onset and periodicity of sounds faithfully (Zhao and Wu, 2001; Zhang and Kelly, 2006).

The nuclei of the lateral lemniscus are particularly well developed in echo-locating bats: the reason may be that the location of echoes from small prey targets (such as moths) is a highly demanding task of temporal processing. Intensive studies in these animals have revealed that the VNLL is a major source of synchronized inhibition in the inferior colliculus and therefore plays an important role in temporal analysis in this nucleus (Huffman and Covey, 1995).

As anatomists at the University of Salamanca have discovered, there is also one unique organizational feature of the VNLL: it has a concentric, helical organization with about 7–8 turns (Merchan and Berbel, 1996; see Fig. 11.10). As we will see in Chapter 11, this remarkable structure may play an important role in the temporal analysis not only of pitch but also of harmony.

6.7   Inferior colliculus

6.7.1   Functional organization

En route to the cortex, almost all auditory information from the brainstem has to pass through the main auditory nucleus of the midbrain, the inferior colliculus. Therefore, as manifold as the processing in the brainstem may be, the inferior colliculus has to take care of its results. Some acoustic information is transmitted to the inferior colliculus from the olivary nuclei, but a major part of the information stream from the CN bypasses the olivary nuclei and reaches the inferior colliculus directly. Stellate, fusiform and giant cells all send their axons directly to make contact with cells in the inferior colliculus on the opposite side, but there are also some projections to the inferior colliculus on the same side.

The inferior colliculus consists of several anatomically and functionally different parts. During conferences on auditory processing, electrophysiologists and neuroanatomists have on occasion had hot disputes about the right way to define the number and boundaries of the different substructures – but they do agree that the main part of the inferior colliculus, known as the 'central nucleus', is the part that receives the majority of the ascending inputs.

6.7.2   Tonotopy in the midbrain

The central nucleus retains tonotopy, the orderly spatial representation of frequency in the cochlea. The tonotopy in the inferior colliculus was first demonstrated in cats by Michael Merzenich and Miriam Reid from the University of California in San Francisco (1974). They found a continuous dorsal to ventral gradient of neuronal CFs; neurons in dorsal parts of the central nucleus respond best to low frequencies, while those in the ventral part prefer high frequencies.

As far as we know, this arrangement holds for all mammals, including humans, and at first view one might assume that there must be a continuous spatial organization along the dorso-ventral tonotopic gradient. Detailed studies, however, have revealed that this is not the case. The structure of the central nucleus stands out as a discontinuous laminar organization composed of input fibres and the dendrites of its principal neurons. Scientists have distinguished about 30 discrete, parallel 'fibro-dendritic laminae' that have a thickness of 0.1–0.2 mm in the cat (Rockel and Jones, 1973; Oliver and Morest, 1984); and are oriented approximately at right angles (orthogonal) to the dorsal-to-ventral frequency gradient (Figs. 6.13, 6.14a). The two major cell types in the inferior colliculus, the disc-shaped and the stellate cells, send their axons roughly orthogonally across the neuronal laminae to reach the auditory part of the thalamus (medial geniculate body). While disc-shaped cells keep their dendrites mostly in a particular lamina, the dendrites of stellate cells may cross many laminae (Fig. 6.13).

A quite efficient way to demonstrate details of the tonotopic organization in the inferior colliculus is provided by the 2-deoxyglucose method. In such experiments neurons that are activated by an acoustic stimulus take up radioactive glucose. X-ray films can then be exposed to radioactive slices obtained from the sectioned brain.

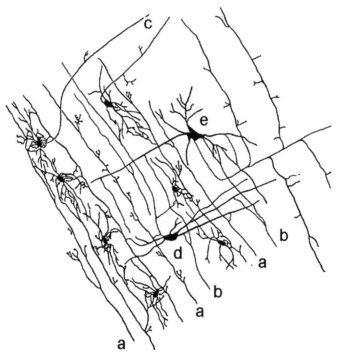

Fig. 6.13   As shown above for the cat, the input fibres **(a, b)** of the central part of the inferior colliculus are organized in about 30 laminae (only two are shown in the figure). The nucleus contains two cell types: disc-shaped and stellate. Disc-shaped cells receive their input from a narrow range of afferents and send their axons **(c)** perpendicular to the neuronal laminae, to the thalamus. The dendrites of stellate cells **(d, e)** cross many laminae and therefore receive many inputs (modified from Oliver and Morest, 1984).

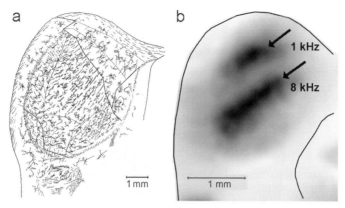

a   b

1 kHz

8 kHz

1 mm   1 mm

Fig. 6.14   **(a)** The central nucleus of the inferior colliculus is characterized by about 30 fibro-dendritic laminae. The lines in the section through the left inferior colliculus of a cat delineate subnuclei which can be distinguished by anatomical criteria (modified from Oliver, 2005). **(b)** Metabolic labelling (2-deoxyglucose method) of neurons in the inferior colliculus of a gerbil following acoustic stimulation with two tones (1 kHz and 8 kHz, 65 dB SPL; modified from Langner, 2004).

In Fig. 6.14b the resulting dark bands along the fibro-dendritic laminae in an inferior colliculus slice indicate areas where neurons have reacted to the acoustic stimuli and therefore accumulated radioactivity. The size and orientation of these bands correspond to the laminar organization (Fig. 6.14a). In the example shown here the labelled bands are quite broad because the tones were loud enough to activate neurons in several adjacent laminae.

6.7.3   The fine structure of tonotopy

The laminae in the inferior colliculus are still often addressed as 'isofrequency planes', implying that the thousands of neurons of a given lamina would all share a preference for the same frequency. This would at best be a strange concept. There are about 3500 inner hair cells which are all tuned to different frequencies. Consequently, assuming a homogeneous distribution of input fibres reaching the ~30 laminae of the inferior colliculus, there should be information from about 120 different hair cells in each lamina, which should therefore represent certain frequency bands.

This raises the question as to whether there might also be an orderly tonotopic arrangement along a given lamina. To answer this question Christoph Schreiner (University of California, San Francisco) and myself measured the CF of neurons in the central nucleus of the cat. We found that the CFs did not increase continuously along the tonotopic gradient, but in steps (Schreiner and Langner, 1997). Moreover, our investigations in cats revealed a fine structure of tonotopic organization in neuronal laminae, orthogonal to the main frequency gradient of the inferior colliculus (Fig. 6.15). In each 'frequency-band laminae', the CFs of the neurons varied systematically over a small range of frequencies (less than one-third of an octave). Our findings were supported also in the inferior colliculus of rats (Malmierca *et al.*, 2008).

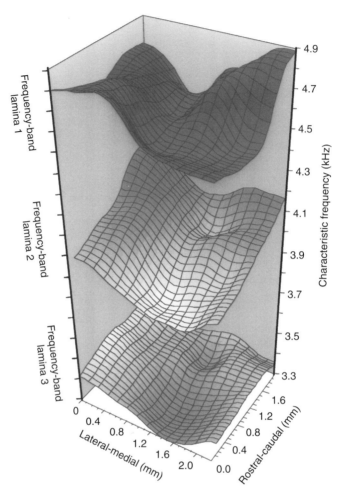

Fig. 6.15 The fine structure of tonotopy in the inferior colliculus. Each of the three selected
frequency-band laminae in the inferior colliculus of the cat is aligned orthogonal to the main
frequency gradient of the inferior colliculus. The CFs of single and small groups of neurons
in the laminae vary systematically over a small range of frequencies (one-third of an
octave). Note that the *x*- and *y*-axis contain spatial coordinates while the *z*-axis is frequency
(CFs of neurons; from Schreiner and Langner, 1997).

6.7.4   Tonotopic fine structure and critical bands

The spatial relationship of a laminated anatomical structure, and a specific distribution of
functional properties within and across laminae, allows for the simplification of complicated processing tasks. Probably the central nucleus of the inferior colliculus is where
the auditory system generates the so-called critical bands (Ehret and Merzenich, 1985;
Egorova and Ehret, 2008). Critical bands or critical bandwidths have been a favourite
topic of psycho-acousticians for some decades, since it was shown that somehow the
auditory system is able to integrate spectral energy over bands of frequency in order to

judge loudness or to detect signals in noise (Fletcher and Munson, 1933; Zwicker *et al.*, 1957). If the bandwidth of a masking noise is smaller than the critical bandwidth, it is less effective in obscuring (masking) a test tone.

As intriguing as this fine structure of frequency organization may be, it is only the tip of the iceberg. We will hear more about the complex neuronal machinery of the inferior colliculus in Chapters 8 and 9, although – for the sake of brevity – I will not discuss the mapping of binaural information, nor the processing of other signal features such as amplitude, duration or frequency modulation in the inferior colliculus. In Chapter 10 we will instead concentrate on the spatial representation of pitch information that, in addition to the results of the cochlear frequency analysis, is mapped on the neuronal laminae of the inferior colliculus.

6.8   Thalamus, the gateway to the cortex

The central nucleus of the inferior colliculus projects to the next processing centre of the auditory system, the medial geniculate body in the thalamus (MGB). The thalamus is generally considered to be the gateway to the cortex, as virtually all sensory information has to pass through it. There are still many more questions than answers about the neuronal processing (not only) in this part of the brain. Probably the MGB is a kind of relay station where – in cooperation with the adjacent thalamic reticular nucleus, cortical processing centres and the limbic system – decisions are made concerning which information may pass through and which should be enhanced or suppressed (Kimura *et al.*, 2007). For example, neurons in the thalamus are probably in charge of alerting the cortex and providing relevant information when our name is uttered amid the noise of a cocktail party.

The MGB by itself is a complicated structure with several subdivisions but, as one might expect, its main part – known as the ventral division – has a tonotopic organization. Moreover, there is also evidence for a tonotopic fine structure in the ventral division that seems to parallel the layered tonotopic organization of the inferior colliculus (Cetas *et al.*, 2001). In addition, although this has yet to be determined, there should be a spatial representation of pitch, because the spatial pitch information which arises in the midbrain also finally arrives at the cortex (see Chapter 10).

6.9   The cortex

6.9.1   Tonotopy in the cortex

All relevant information in our auditory system will finally be transmitted to the last station in the actual hearing pathway – the auditory cortex. This processing centre lies in posterior regions of the cortical hemispheres, on the superior plane of the temporal lobe. Similar to other sensory cortices, it is not a uniform single structure but can be subdivided into several areas including what is now known as the primary auditory field (AI).

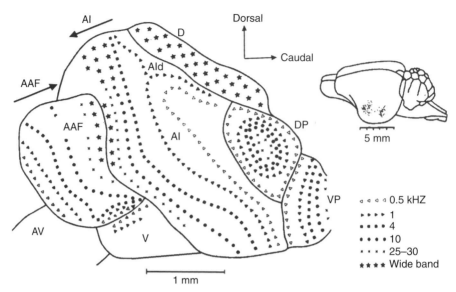

Fig. 6.16   This scheme of the frequency organization of the gerbil's auditory cortex was derived by pooling the data from electrophysiological recordings in nine animals. Boundaries of the different physiologically defined fields are indicated by continuous lines (modified from Thomas *et al.*, 1993).

Whether or not these areas are tonotopically organized was disputed for many years (Ehret, 1997). This is especially astonishing as the first evidence for a tonotopy in the cortex had already been obtained in the first half of the last century by C. G. Woolsey and E. M. Walzl in the cat (1942) and by Archie Tunturi in the dog (1944).

An example from a more recent and detailed electrophysiological study is given in Fig. 6.16. It shows the various tonotopic organizations of several different auditory cortical fields in gerbils. The organization of the gerbil auditory cortex is highly elaborate; the parcellation into fields is as complex as in cats or primates. Adjacent to the large primary auditory field (AI), additional tonotopic representations were found. For example, the tonotopic organization of the anterior auditory field (AAF) is a mirror image of that in AI (indicated by arrows), while the dorso-posterior field (DP) is concentrically organized with best frequencies increasing from the periphery to the centre. Besides frequency, a variety of sound parameters (e.g. bandwidth of tuning, binaural sensitivity and intensity) are spatially and temporally represented in these different cortical fields (Schreiner and Mendelson, 1990). The map for periodicity pitch is especially simple, with pitch increasing along a constant gradient roughly at a right angle to the tonotopic gradient (see Figs. 10.8–10.13).

6.9.2   Wernicke's area

The processing of acoustic information does not end in the fields of the auditory cortex. Hearing information has to be compared to and combined with information

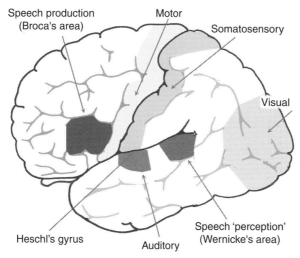

Speech production
(Broca's area)   Motor
                                          Somatosensory

                                              Visual

Heschl's gyrus   Speech 'perception'
                          Auditory   (Wernicke's area)

Fig. 6.17   The auditory cortex is located below the cortical area for the sensory processing of touch and
other somatosensory signals. It extends further into the depth of Heschl's gyrus. Speech signals
are received and processed in Wernicke's area. Close to the motor cortex, the centre for the
coordination of movements, lies Broca's area, the centre for speech production.

from other sensory systems. This allows us to draw the right conclusions from the
sensory input and to elicit the right motor responses. On one side of the cortex (the left
side in most right-handers and the right side in some left-handers) is an area known as
the Wernicke area (named after its discoverer, the German neuropathologist Carl
Wernicke, 1848–1905).

Because Wernicke's area is specialized for the processing of auditory speech signals
(Wernicke, 1874), it makes sense that this cortical area lies in the temporal lobe close to
the primary auditory fields (Fig. 6.17). Again, nobody knows exactly what the millions
of cells in this centre are doing, although it seems clear that they are involved in our
understanding of speech. If we learn a second language, the size of Wernicke's area
increases and some parts are devoted exclusively to the new language, while patients
with infarcts in this area suffer from an impairment of speech comprehension
(Wernicke's aphasia).

6.9.3   Broca's area

There is yet another area in the brain devoted to language, but in this area the neurons
become activated when we are speaking or singing. This motor speech centre is in the
frontal cortex, and is known as Broca's area (named after its discoverer, the French
physician Pierre Paul Broca, 1824–1880). In contrast to Wernicke's area, it is active in
speech production rather than in speech comprehension.

It makes sense that this area lies close to the motor centre of the cortex, where
commands for the muscles involved in speech production are generated (Fig. 6.17).

People with deficits in Broca's area can understand speech but have difficulties in producing a normal fluent pattern of speech (Broca's aphasia or expressive aphasia). Although words can be uttered they may have no meaning for the listener as the language of the patients is disjointed and their sentence construction and intonation poor.

6.9.4   'What- and where-streams'

As mentioned above, there has already been a pre-selection of information at the level of the thalamus. The cortex, therefore, does not receive all the information which reaches our processing centres at lower levels. This is advantageous, because it helps us to concentrate on relevant information and to neglect the irrelevant. As one would expect, however, this may also result in situations where we dismiss certain aspects of our environment that nevertheless may turn out to be important. On the other hand, although the activation of the auditory cortex is necessary for conscious hearing, it was demonstrated to be insufficient; conscious perception also needs simultaneous and, it seems, synchronized activity in the prefrontal cortex.

Quite appropriately, neuroscientists have demonstrated so-called 'what- and where-streams' of processing in the human cortex and in that of non-human primates (Rauschecker and Tian, 2000; Rauschecker and Scott, 2009). It is the task of these 'cortical streams' to pass information from the back of our brain to the front. Dorsal areas of the cortex seem to be devoted mainly to answering the question of where certain visual or auditory information that reaches our body comes from. They are also concerned about their temporal order while others, more at the lower and lateral side of the cortex, have the task of determining what kind of information it may be. It is conceivable that these processing streams must be essential for speech understanding and speech production.

This intriguing finding has led to a clearer understanding of the function as well as potential dysfunction of certain parts of the cortex. Nevertheless, nobody really knows what the billions of cortical nerve cells with their trillions of intricate connections are really doing. Certainly, we are still missing essential pieces of information before we can even start to understand our own brains. In my opinion, what is lacking is a deeper understanding of the dynamic processes that connect cortical areas, as well as subcortical structures in the thalamus and the brainstem, to a great extent by means of synchronized oscillations (see Chapter 12).

6.9.5   A music centre?

Another interesting property of the auditory cortex is the lateralization of musical processing. Many experiments have demonstrated that music is processed predominantly in the right cortex. For example, when the right side of the brain is anaesthetized, patients can still speak but lose their ability to sing. It is remarkable that this lateralization is more prominent in non-musicians than in musicians.

Functional imaging techniques have shown that trained musicians make more extensive use of both sides of their brain. They also have stronger connections between both cortical sides through the corpus callosum, the fibre tract that connects the two sides of the cortex. Finally, in the frontal part of the brain there seems to be a cortical field devoted to music – this area was found to be most strongly activated with musical stimulation (Zatorre and Samson, 1991; Liégeois-Chauvel *et al.*, 1998).

7   Periodicity coding in the brainstem

7.1   Periodicity coding in the auditory nerve

7.1.1   Temporal coding

As we know from the previous chapter, a pure tone activates a certain place on the basilar membrane maximally, and hair cells at this place code the frequency of that signal by their position along the membrane. However, we also know that this labelled line coding, or 'place information', alone is not sufficient to explain the acuity of our perception and that the central auditory system obviously must make use of additional information that is supplied by the temporal firing patterns of the nerve fibres.

We also saw that the limited frequency resolution of our cochlea is actually advantageous for the temporal analysis of – for example – a harmonic sound. When its frequency range is sufficiently broad, neural responses in many frequency channels will be elicited by a waveform that is a superposition of harmonic components of the harmonic sound. As a consequence, hair cells signal the presence and intensity of the harmonics to which they are tuned to the central auditory system, but they also transmit temporal information about this superposition. Because all the components of a harmonic sound are integer multiples of its fundamental frequency, the periodicity of their superposition will correspond to that of the fundamental frequency (or a multiple thereof, if certain harmonics are missing). As a result, the fundamental of a harmonic sound is encoded by the temporal discharge patterns of auditory nerve fibres even if it is physically absent. This explains why, after a corresponding temporal analysis in the central auditory system, we are able to perceive the pitch of what Schouten called the 'missing fundamental'.

If the fundamental can be coded in the auditory nerve, the question arises as to how the corresponding temporal information is decoded in the nervous system and how the properties of the nerve and the neurons in the brain contribute to this temporal analysis. We will see that auditory nerve fibres exhibit low response diversity when compared to neurons in the cochlear nucleus (CN) and higher auditory centres. Nevertheless, fibres which are tuned to the same frequency may differ in ways that are quite useful for the subsequent temporal analysis.

At least two classes of nerve fibres can be distinguished on the basis of their response thresholds and spontaneous rate of spike discharges (Liberman, 1978; Kim and Molnar, 1979). Fibres of the first class (~80%) have response thresholds that are close to the hearing threshold (low-threshold fibres). They also have a high spontaneous activity, i.e. they fire 20 or more spikes per second and, most important in our context, show prominent responses to envelope periodicities. Fibres of the second class (~20%) have high thresholds and low spontaneous rates (high-threshold fibres). Their coding of envelope periodicities is less precise and they put more emphasis on the temporal fine structure of a signal (Horst *et al.*, 1985). Obviously, the auditory system starts to separate the envelope and the carrier of a sound signal as the first step of temporal processing.

The previous chapter showed that auditory nerve fibres synchronize to frequencies up to about 5 kHz. This so-called 'upper limit of phase coupling' basically reflects the natural limitation of temporal precision of all kinds of neurons. Nevertheless, it has been demonstrated that auditory nerve fibres can synchronize to periodic envelopes with modulation frequencies even higher than 5 kHz (Palmer, 1982). On the other hand, neurons in processing centres below the auditory midbrain are quite unselective for periodic signals. Accordingly, all auditory nerve fibres behave simply like low-pass filters for modulation frequencies (Fig. 7.1); their modulation-transfer functions (MTFs; see Box 7.1) do not show significant preferences for a certain modulation frequency as long as they are below a certain upper limit (cut-off frequency; Møller, 1976; Javel, 1980; Frisina *et al.*, 1990; Kim *et al.*, 1990). This upper limit increases with the absolute bandwidth of the tuning curves of the fibres, which on this part increases with their centre frequency (Palmer, 1982), while their cut-off frequency always stays below about 1.5 kHz (Joris and Yin, 1992). Since the average activity of the nerve fibres does not show significant preferences for a certain modulation frequency, it is necessary to analyse their temporal response patterns in order to extract information about the modulation of acoustic signals. This is the task of periodicity processing in the auditory brainstem, including the auditory midbrain.

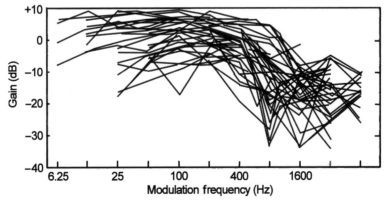

Fig. 7.1   The modulation-transfer functions (MTFs) of cochlear nerve fibres, measured in the guinea pig, are typical for mammals. The gain, plotted on the *y*-axis, is the ratio of the modulation depth (see Fig. 2.6) of the response to that of the stimulus. As a total the fibres display a low-pass characteristic with a cut-off frequency at about 800 Hz, but some response modulation remains even at modulation frequencies around 5 kHz (from Palmer, 1982).

BOX 7.1 The modulation-transfer function (MTF)

It is useful to distinguish between two types of MTFs which indicate how neurons respond to different modulation frequencies. The synchronization MTF shows the average synchronization and the rate-MTF the rate of the neuronal response to a particular carrier frequency modulated with different frequencies (Rees and Møller, 1983; Reimer, 1987; Langner and Schreiner, 1988). If such an MTF has a single distinguishable maximum it is called a 'band-pass MTF' and the maximum is called the 'best modulation frequency' (BMF). Neurons with *low-pass* characteristics respond to all modulation frequencies below a certain maximal value; neurons with *high-pass* characteristics respond to all modulation frequencies above a certain minimal value; and those with *band reject* characteristics respond to modulation frequencies above and below a certain modulation range.

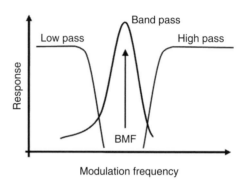

Fig. 7.1.1

7.1.2   Intensity effects

The temporal coding of an amplitude-modulated (AM) signal by a low-threshold nerve fibre depends on the signal intensity (Fig. 7.2). If the modulation frequency is sufficiently high, the spectral distance between the AM components may be comparable to the width of the tuning curve of the fibre. As a result, depending on the intensity of the AM signal, either the spike pattern generated by the fibre could contain information about the signal modulation or, alternatively, the sidebands are suppressed and only the carrier frequency remains encoded (Delgutte, 1980). If the signal is close enough to the threshold, the nerve fibre can even resolve the carrier frequency. In contrast, at a medium level, the three AM components may be within the response area of the fibre and the modulation would be discernible in the period histograms (see Fig. 7.2, right side).

At the highest intensity, low-threshold fibres show still another effect of modulation coding. In contrast to high-threshold fibres they can only increase their activity over a quite limited dynamic range (see Figs 7.6, 7.7). This is called the *saturation effect* and limits the coding capability of low-threshold fibres to a dynamic range of 30–40 dB above their threshold. Above this intensity the response to the modulation is

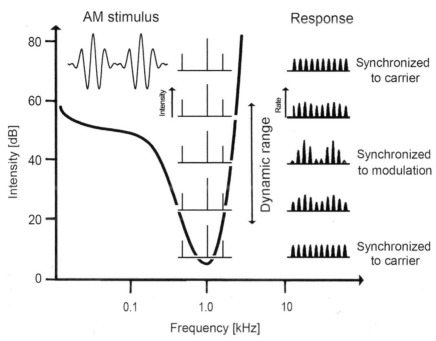

Fig. 7.2   The response of a hypothetical low-threshold nerve fibre is modulated if the intensity of the signal is in its dynamic range (here 20–40 dB). The carrier frequency will be resolved either at low intensities, when the sidebands of the amplitude modulated tone are filtered out (bottom) or at high intensities, when the fibre is saturated. It does not code the modulation (top), because it does not differentiate between low and high modulation amplitudes anymore.

progressively weakened until it resembles that elicited by the carrier alone (Evans and Palmer, 1980; Horst *et al.*, 1990). In summary, the carrier frequency can not only be resolved at low intensities when the sidebands fall out of the tuning curve of the fibre, but also at high intensities when it is saturated.

Such restraining effects of intensity on temporal coding have been demonstrated in the auditory nerve fibres of many animals (Javel, 1980). However, there are several effects which do compensate for these constraints of temporal coding. For example, since the fibres have a dynamic range of 40 dB and the thresholds of different fibres cover a range of another 40 dB, signals are represented in total in the auditory nerve over a large intensity range of 80 dB or even more (Horst *et al.*, 1986).

7.1.3   Population coding and lateral suppression

It is essential for periodicity coding that – as long as the sound intensity is in a physiological range – there will always be many nerve fibres activated in their dynamic range (see Figs 7.6, 7.7; Bahmer and Langner, 2009). When the intensity of an AM signal increases, cells which are tuned to the carrier or adjacent frequencies will be more and more saturated (see above). In addition, an increasing population of fibres will respond which are tuned to other frequencies and therefore still have unsaturated responses (Palmer, 1982; Shivapuja *et al.*, 1990).

Moreover, there are other effects that may also counteract the saturation effect (Sachs and Kiang, 1968). For example, a moderately weak response of a fibre may be suppressed by activity in adjacent frequency ranges (lateral suppression). Taken together, these mechanisms ensure that – in spite of the limitations imposed by the physiology of the single cell – in a large population of nerve fibres temporal information about modulated signals is reliably encoded over a very large intensity range.

7.1.4   Temporal coding of vowels

An essential contribution to our understanding of temporal information coding in the auditory nerve comes from studies which used natural and synthetic vowels as stimuli (Sachs and Young, 1979; Young and Sachs, 1979; Reale and Geisler, 1980; Sinex and Geisler, 1983; Delgutte and Kiang, 1984). As described in Chapter 2, vowels are harmonic signals generated by periodic vibrations of our vocal cords and filtered by resonances in the mouth (see Fig. 2.9).

Nerve fibres which are tuned to a frequency near a formant frequency (resonance maxima) show little or no response modulation corresponding to the fundamental (Fig. 7.3). Instead, they are phase-coupled to the formant frequency or to an adjacent harmonic that falls into their response area, provided its intensity is higher than that of other neighbouring frequency components (Horst *et al.*, 1990). Due to lateral suppression (see Section 7.1.3), the strongest frequency component in the response area of a fibre may even suppress the response to the weaker components (Javel, 1980). As a consequence, the temporal fine structure of auditory nerve responses may carry information about individual harmonics of vowels, in particular about those close to the formants (Young and Sachs, 1979; Delgutte, 1980; Miller and Sachs, 1984).

The coding of harmonics at or close to the formants obviously must be important for the identification of vowels. The complementary aspect is the coding of its fundamental frequency or pitch. The higher harmonics of a vowel superpose increasingly on the basilar membrane and generate modulations corresponding to the fundamental period of a vowel (see Fig. 4.2). The responses of many nerve fibres are therefore modulated with the period of the fundamental and thus carry temporal information about the pitch of a vowel to the neurons of the cochlear nucleus (long arrows in Fig. 7.3).

7.2   Periodicity coding in the cochlear nucleus

7.2.1   Faithful synchronization

Wever's volley principle (see Fig. 6.9) shows that the synchronized activities of populations of auditory nerve fibres may encode pure tones as well as periodic envelopes of harmonic and modulated signals up to about 5 kHz. The nerve fibres transfer this temporal information, distributed over many frequency channels, exclusively to the

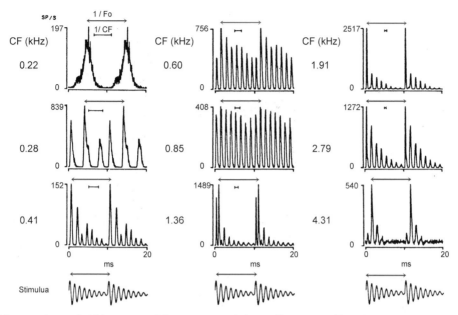

Fig. 7.3 Nine period histograms of the responses of nine auditory nerve fibres (0.22 < CF < 4.31 kHz) to vowel-like sounds (as indicated at the bottom; fundamental: 100 Hz; single formant at 800 Hz; 60 dB SPL). Note that the envelope period of the signal (1/Fo) is coded by all neurons (long arrows), but in particular by those with low and high CFs. However, fibres with a CF around 0.8 kHz represent predominantly the formant frequency (modified from Delgutte, 1980).

CN. For a periodicity analysis to take place in the central auditory system, it is essential that the temporal information transferred by the nerve is somehow preserved in this nucleus. It is, nevertheless, also modified in characteristic ways and there is a significant diversity in periodicity coding among its different types of neurons.

It has been known for decades that even single neurons in the CN can code envelope periodicities, at least up to 800 Hz or even 1000 Hz (Glattke, 1969; Vater, 1982) and different methods of systems analysis have been used to investigate their temporal response properties (Møller, 1972). Nevertheless, it came as a surprise to many auditory scientists that in the processing step from the nerve to the CN, temporal information is not only nicely preserved but often even strongly enhanced (Rhode and Greenberg, 1994).

Aage Møller was the first to systematically exploit modulated tone or noise carriers in order to determine period histograms and MTFs of CN neurons (Møller, 1974a, 1974b, 1976). First, he found in neurons of the rat CN that the dynamic range (see Figs. 7.6, 7.7) for modulation coding is often greater than in the auditory nerve; the same holds for their dynamic range for pure tones. Moreover, Møller's results showed that the modulation of the discharge rate of neurons (elicited by the modulation of the stimulus) may be much larger than the modulation of the acoustic stimulus itself. He concluded that neurons in the CN provide clear information about the rate and magnitude of the modulation of the sound intensity or signal envelope.

The response modulation of neurons is enhanced even when the stimulus intensity is 60 dB above the threshold of the neuron. In comparison, efficient modulation coding in auditory nerve fibres usually requires that the stimulus intensity is less than 30 dB above the threshold of the fibres (see Fig. 7.2). In other words, efficient modulation coding in the CN is possible at a sound intensity at least 1000 times higher than intensities which may be efficient in the nerve.

As seen above, the MTFs of the nerve fibres have mainly low-pass characteristics (Fig. 7.1), i.e. neurons respond alike to all low frequencies below an upper limit. For neurons in the cochlear nucleus this is also true at low intensities, but at higher intensities they are often tuned, although only quite broadly, to a particular frequency (see Figs. 7.7, 7.9; Frisina *et al.*, 1985, 1990). In contrast, except at very high stimulus levels or large modulation depths, amplitude modulations are reproduced with high fidelity in the intervals of neuronal responses (Hirsch and Gibson, 1976; Møller and Rees, 1986). The upper frequency limit for this kind of faithful temporal encoding is approximately 1000 pHz (Møller, 1972).

7.2.2   Diversity of periodicity coding

In Chapter 6, response diversity has been characterized by the temporal responses to pure tones, but – important for subsequent central periodicity analysis – different cell types in the CN are also characterized by the way they encode periodicity information (Frisina *et al.*, 1990). For example, the ability to synchronize to AM signals is quite different in different neuronal types. Interestingly, the more their responses to pure tones differ from that of an auditory nerve fibre, the more they are able to synchronize to modulated sounds (Frisina *et al.*, 1985). Moreover, primary-like, onset and chopper neurons differ greatly in their abilities to encode modulations at higher intensities; the synchronization of both onset and chopper neurons is even better than that of the auditory nerve (see Figs. 7.7, 7.9).

7.2.3   Bushy cells

The giant input synapses of bushy cells allow these neurons to code temporal information with high precision. Their response properties, including their synchronization to periodic signals, closely resemble those of the auditory nerve cells and therefore are called 'primary-like'. Accordingly, they also preserve the envelope periodicities of harmonic sounds as well as of amplitude modulations (Moore and Cashin, 1976; Caspary *et al.*, 1977; Rupert *et al.*, 1977). As a result of the convergence of a (small) number of nerve fibres they may sum up the common periodicities of their input fibres and signal amplitude modulations even more clearly than the nerve fibres, especially at higher intensities (Frisina *et al.*, 1985).

As we saw in Chapter 6, bushy cells project to the olivary nuclei (Warr, 1982), which are involved primarily, if not exclusively, in binaural information processing. Because of this, one might be justified in concluding that bushy cells are of minor importance for the neuronal processing of acoustic patterns and, especially, for periodicity analysis (Frisina *et al.*, 1990). As their response patterns are barely distinguishable from those of the nerve fibres, their function may mostly be to amplify and enhance the timing of their input and transfer the result to the olivary nuclei where it can be compared with information impinging from the opposite side. Obviously the functional role of these neurons is to provide information for binaural localization and thus belongs to those aspects of auditory processing which are outside the main scope of this book.

On the other hand, this does not mean that periodicity information is useless for acoustic localization. We are able to evaluate the difference of either the intensities or the arrival times of the sounds at our two ears. A tiny difference in arrival times (<1 ms) indicates that the sound source is closer to one ear than to the other. When the sound is located to the front of us, we are able to distinguish differences in arrival times as small as 10 µs (Klumpp and Eady, 1956).

In addition, since our head creates an acoustic shadow when exposed to sound waves, small intensity differences are created between the two ears. For pure tones above 1 kHz, the acoustic wavelengths are comparable to, or smaller than, our head size, which makes the arrival times of waves at our ears ambiguous; in this situation intensity cues are all that remain for the task of localization. In summary, the frequency limit of about 1 kHz for temporal localization is correct only for pure tones, but does not hold for complex signals and therefore for most of our acoustic environment. For these signals we can use the time difference between the arrival of modulations at the left and right ears for localization. The only condition is that the modulation periods are larger than about 1 ms (modulation frequency <1 kHz). This is the reason why the precise temporal coding of periodicity by bushy cells in the CN may be important for sound localization.

7.2.4   Octopus cells

The octopus cells (onset neurons) which lie in close proximity to stellate cells in the ventral CN (see Figs 6.10, 7.4) were first described in the 1960s (Pfeiffer, 1966). At high frequencies they 'fire' a single action potential with a short delay after tone onset (Figs.6.11c, 7.6b). However, they behave quite differently when the stimulus has a periodicity to which they are able to synchronize (Figs. 7.5, 7.6c, d). In 1970, Aage Møller recorded from onset neurons in the rat, although at that time he called them 'transient units'. It is still intriguing to see how such neurons respond with a single precisely timed action potential, not only to a single sound click but to every click in a series up to a certain periodicity (Fig. 7.5a). Above this signal period their response strength drops sharply (Fig. 7.5b). For some octopus cells the upper limit of synchronization is at least as high as 800 Hz.

Because octopus cells integrate over quite a large frequency range (Fig. 7.6a), it is quite unlikely that they can contribute significantly to spectral analysis and frequency representation. They simply can't 'tell' much about the difference between frequencies. In contrast, their anatomical arrangement and connections make them quite suitable for the summation of temporally coinciding impulses on their many input fibres. Their large dendrites extend over large arrays of auditory nerve fibres, which are especially

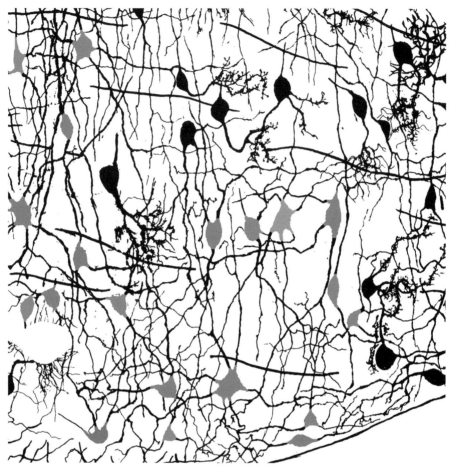

Fig. 7.4   Octopus cells (black) and stellate cells (grey) in the PVCN are in close proximity. Note that the applied Golgi method labels only a small fraction of the cells that are actually present (the shading of stellate cells modified; from Lorente de Nó, 1981, fig. 4.2).

concentrated in their vicinity. As a result the octopus cells receive their input from many nerve fibres; it was estimated that they make contacts with 50 or even more fibres (see Fig. 6.12; Willott and Bross, 1990). These fibres arise from large areas of the cochlea and, as a result, while octopus cells are not very useful for frequency discrimination, they are very sensitive to amplitude fluctuations which arise in the frequency range of their inputs.

Octopus cells do not only respond to the onset of a tone (or click); they may also synchronize in response to low-frequency pure tones below about 1.5 kHz (Godfrey *et al.*, 1975; Bourk, 1976; Britt and Starr, 1976; Rhode and Smith, 1986). Even for frequencies far from their characteristic frequency, they may precisely fire one spike at a certain phase of each stimulus period (Fig. 7.6c, d; Greenberg, 1988). Moreover, they show reliable synchronized responses to AM signals and encode the fundamental frequency of complex sounds with exceptional temporal precision (Rhode, 1994,

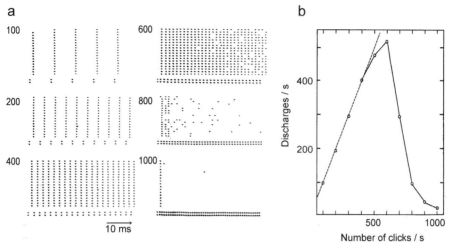

Fig. 7.5   **(a)** The 'point plots' of the responses of an onset neuron ('transient unit') in the CN of the rat show that this neuron type may synchronize to high repetition rates of clicks. It 'fires' a single action potential to every click in a series, up to a rate of at least 600 Hz (each dot stands for an action potential). The repetition rate in clicks per second is indicated by the inserted numbers and the individual clicks are shown by the double dots below each recording sequence (click duration 30 ms). **(b)** The average number of action potentials per second as a function of repetition rate. The dashed line shows a one-to-one relationship between stimulus and response. In the example shown, the response strength drops sharply above a rate of 600 clicks per second (modified from Møller, 1970).

1998; Oertel *et al.*, 2000). They actually show the strongest phase-locking to amplitude modulations of all neurons in the CN (Frisina *et al.*, 1985).

Furthermore, octopus cells by far exceed the synchronization, the maximum firing rates and the gain (amplification) of modulation of their auditory nerve inputs (Rhode and Smith, 1986; Oertel *et al.*, 2000). While auditory nerve fibres code amplitude modulations only over a small intensity range of 40 dB, some octopus cells (and also stellate cells; see below) maintain their ability to synchronize responses over a much larger intensity range of at least 90 dB (Fig. 7.7). Again, the reason is probably that octopus cells receive a large number of convergent inputs (see above) and act as precise coincidence detectors. For this purpose they benefit from an extremely fast potassium channel which is activated at a low threshold and contributes to a very short membrane time constant of about 0.2 ms (Golding *et al.*, 1999; Bal and Oertel, 2001; Rothmans and Manis, 2003a). The temporal coding properties of octopus cells suggest that they play an important role in periodicity analysis and the perception of pitch. Their coding properties are perfect for the detection of amplitude modulations that are synchronous over more or less broad extents of the basilar membrane. Since they are able to detect transients of sound and may respond very quickly to quite variable signals, it is likely that they also contribute to attention, and trigger alarm reactions such as the so-called startle or shock response.

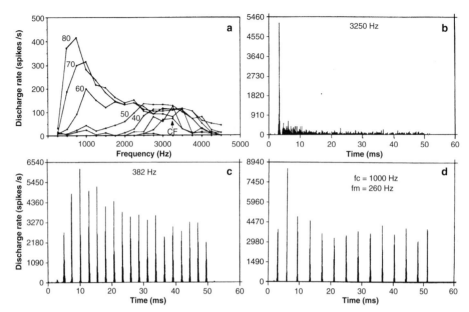

Fig. 7.6   (a) Responses of an onset neuron in the CN of the cat to pure tones at different intensities reveal a very broad tuning over a frequency range of more than two octaves. (b) The response to a tone at its characteristic frequency (CF) is dominated by a strong on-response. (c) In contrast, low-frequency tones elicit a highly synchronized response during the whole stimulation. (d) The same holds for AM signals, for example a carrier of 1000 Hz modulated by a frequency of 260 Hz (modified from Greenberg, 1988).

7.2.5   Stellate cells

In Section 6.3 stellate cells were described as a large and important group of neurons in the CN. T-stellate cells ('chopper neurons') respond with sustained or transient oscillations to various kinds of stimuli (Rhode *et al.*, 1983b; Langner, 1992; Oertel *et al.*, 2011). They project to the midbrain and – according to the periodicity model presented in Section 9.4 – activate coincidence cells that are involved in periodicity analysis. On the other hand, D-stellate cells, which are also known as 'onset choppers', restrict their contribution to auditory processing to the CN on both sides of the brain.

Quite in contrast to octopus cells, T-stellate cells receive their input from a very small number (4–6) of auditory nerve fibres with similar characteristic frequencies and, consequently, are only narrowly tuned (Ferragamo *et al.*, 1998). It is astonishing, therefore, that they can synchronize so well to periodic modulations of sound (Figs. 7.8, 7.9; Frisina *et al.*, 1997). This is true for the modulation of tones (amplitude modulations) as well as for envelope modulations reflecting the fundamental frequency of harmonic sounds. Examples of such synchronized responses come from electrophysiological recordings of stellate cells using synthetic vowels as acoustic stimuli (Sachs *et al.*, 1988). In contrast, the phase-locking of stellate cells to pure tones is clearly less precise than that of the primary-like cells.

ON-L

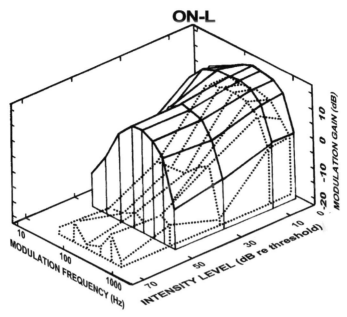

Fig. 7.7   The modulation responses of an octopus cell (onset neuron) and an auditory nerve fibre of the gerbil are characterized in three dimensions: modulation frequency, intensity and modulation gain. The onset neuron (solid lines; CF = 12.0 kHz, modulation depth = 35%) shows a larger modulation gain than the auditory nerve fibre (dotted lines) and also than chopper neurons (see Fig. 7.9). Onset neurons may synchronize their responses over intensity ranges of more than 90 dB (only partly shown for the example above; Frisina *et al.*, 1990).

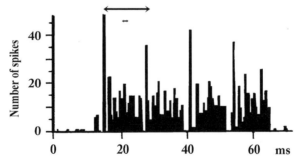

Fig. 7.8   The peri-stimulus time histogram (PSTH) shows the oscillatory response of a chopper neuron (T-stellate cell) in the CN of the gerbil. The stimulus was an amplitude modulation (50 ms duration) with its carrier at the best frequency of the neuron. The *x*-axis represents time with stimulus onset at 10 ms; the *y*-axis represents spike density (spikes/bin). The long arrow indicates the modulation period and the short one the period of the intrinsic oscillations triggered by each modulation wave (modified from Frisina *et al.*, 1997).

Surprisingly, stellate cells – in spite of their intrinsic oscillations – show the best periodicity coding of all neurons in the CN, apart from octopus cells (Frisina *et al.*, 1985, 1990). In response to pure tones, they saturate at only 10–30 dB above threshold, just like auditory nerve fibres (see above). In periodicity coding, however, they

CHOPPER

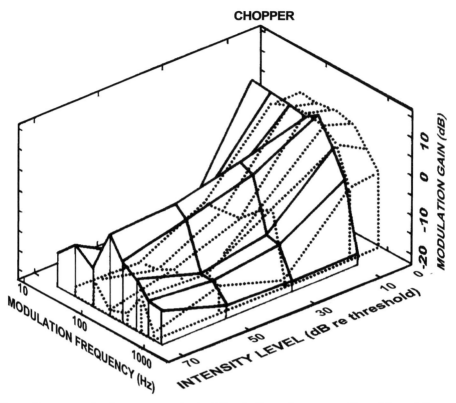

Fig. 7.9   Responses of a chopper neuron in the CN and of an auditory nerve fibre of the gerbil to amplitude modulations (compare Fig. 7.7). The neuron shows a larger modulation gain (solid lines; CF = 9.9 kHz, modulation depth = 35%) than a typical auditory nerve fibre (dotted lines) (from Frisina *et al.*, 1990).

surpass their fibre inputs because they are able to synchronize to modulations, sometimes even up to 90 dB above their response threshold (Bahmer and Langner, 2006a, 2006b, 2007, 2009).

In a similar way to octopus cells, stellate cells also amplify amplitude modulations in their responses to an extent which far surpasses the amplification already observed in the auditory nerve. This amplification even increases with increasing intensity. It is remarkable that, at higher sound levels, stellate cells as well as octopus cells are tuned – although only quite broadly – to certain modulation frequencies (Figs. 7.6, 7.8).

Although stellate cells exceed auditory nerve fibres in synchronization to modulated sounds, their temporal response patterns are actually dominated by their intrinsic oscillations (Fig. 7.8; Frisina *et al.*, 1997). The term 'intrinsic' indicates that their oscillation periods are unrelated to any periods contained in stimulus waveforms (Pfeiffer, 1966; Rhode *et al.*, 1983b; Rouiller and Ryugo, 1984). Accordingly, there seems to be no clear relationship between chopping frequencies and preferred modulation frequencies of stellate cells (Frisina *et al.*, 1990). Instead, if a modulated signal elicits intrinsic oscillations, they tend to be triggered by each single modulation wave (Fig. 7.8).

The questions evoked by the coding properties of stellate cells are a challenge for all models of auditory temporal processing (Langner, 1981, 1985). These questions are: How are intrinsic oscillations triggered? Why are stellate cells, in spite of their narrow frequency tuning, able to code modulations nearly as reliably as the broadly tuned octopus cells? Why do they transform their 'primary-like' input activity into a new oscillating pattern and what does the brain accomplish in making that elaborate transformation? We will address these questions in detail in Chapter 9.

On the basis of intracellular recordings of anatomically defined cells in slices of the CN of the mouse, Ferragamo *et al.* (1998) suggested that T-stellate cells are narrowly tuned because they are activated by only a few auditory nerve fibres. In line with computer simulations (Bahmer and Langner, 2006a, 2006b, 2007, 2009; see also Figs 9.5, 9.6) this suggests that T-stellate cells are connected to each other and excite other stellate cells tuned to similar frequencies. As a result of the positive feedback, the neurons generate intrinsic oscillations.

The circuit raises the question of whether the mutual excitation is self-sustaining and how the oscillation is started and terminated. In Chapter 9, I propose that octopus cells provide the necessary onset triggers for an intrinsic oscillation. Suppression of the oscillations comes from slightly delayed inhibitory inputs from broadly tuned D-stellate cells and other inhibitory interneurons in the DCN (tuberculoventral cells; Wickesberg and Oertel, 1990; Bahmer and Langner, 2007).

7.2.6   Dorsal cochlear nucleus

Many details about the DCN and its constituent neuronal types are quite well known; the diversity of inputs to DCN neurons, their internal connections and their output projections have all been thoroughly investigated. Together with T-stellate cells, principal cells provide the major input to the inferior colliculus, but their targets in the DCN are unknown. We know from Section 6.4 that the systematic spatial projection of the auditory nerve provides a tonotopic frequency organization for its principal cells, the fusiform and the giant cells. Nevertheless, the role of the DCN in auditory processing remains still quite elusive.

While the synchronization to pure tones in principal cells is much less pronounced than that of neurons in the VCN (Goldberg and Brownell, 1973; Rhode and Smith, 1986), they do follow envelope fluctuations of harmonic complexes very reliably, even up to 1200 Hz (Schreiner and Snyder, 1987; Rhode and Greenberg,1994; Zhao and Liang, 1995). Principal cells have several features which underline their special role in periodicity coding. Here are three examples:

(1) Loud noise disturbs the hearing process, as we know from experience, but under these conditions principal cells can actually enhance their periodicity coding over a large range of intensities (Frisina *et al.*, 1994).
(2) It is obvious that it is more difficult for us to detect a weakly than a strongly modulated signal. Principal cells, however, synchronize to even extremely small modulations (2% modulation depth) and, moreover, can increase their synchronization even when the modulation of the signal decreases (Zhao and Liang, 1995).

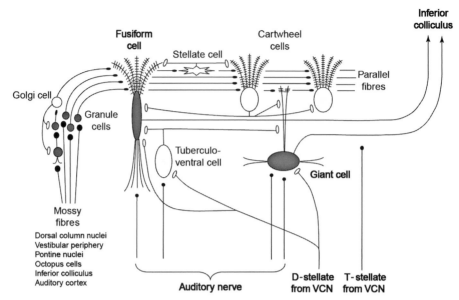

Fig. 7.10   In the DCN auditory nerve fibres innervate the basal dendrites of principal (fusiform and giant) cells, and the inhibitory tuberculoventral cells, all of which are also inhibited by D-stellate cells. Likely sources of terminals in the granule cell region are listed at the lower left of the diagram. Parallel fibres (the axons of granule cells) contact fusiform cells and, to a lesser degree, giant and cartwheel cells, as well as inhibitory interneurons (modified from Oertel and Young, 2004).

(3) Principal cells are highly synchronized to periodic signals up to very high intensities (90 dB SPL) and almost independently of intensity. This led to the conclusion that they code the temporal fine structure of the waveform and not the signal intensity (Zhao and Liang, 1995).

On the basis of such findings it seems justified to interpret the wiring and response properties of DCN neurons in the context of periodicity processing. This is in line with the observation that the arrangement of the superficial layers of the DCN is quite similar to that of the cerebellum, which is known for its temporal processing and delay mechanisms (Oertel and Young, 2004). Naturally, this viewpoint cannot answer all the questions about the DCN and, as is common in science, leads to a bundle of new questions.

Experimental evidence indicates that the responses of principal cells reflect the interaction of multiple excitatory and inhibitory inputs (Fig. 7.10; Parham and Kim, 1995; Oertel and Young, 2004). In order to understand, at least to a certain extent, how this complicated circuit may contribute to the processing of periodic signals, we will start with the first type of inhibitory interneurons, the tuberculoventral cells. These cells receive input from the auditory nerve and are excited by narrowband stimuli (Rhode, 1999; Spirou *et al.*, 1999). As a result, stimuli which are restricted to a narrow frequency range – or are, like formants, very strong in that range – activate these cells. They are then able to inhibit the principal cells (Voigt and Young, 1990; Zhang and Oertel, 1993). However, the tuberculoventral cells on their part are inhibited by D-stellate cells of the VCN (Joris and Smith, 1998).

As we know from above, D-stellate cells (onset choppers) receive input from a wide range of frequencies and synchronize to the onset of signals as well as to the modulations of complex signals. Therefore, the principal cells are released from inhibition after each onset or modulation and are then excited by their direct auditory nerve fibre inputs. Since this does not happen with pure tones (or only at their onsets), they are mostly inhibited by pure tones as well as by narrowband signals. Instead, they prefer broadband signals, which are usually more or less modulated.

As Fig. 7.10 shows, D-stellate cells also directly inhibit the principal cells. Probably this inhibition serves as a kind of reset, which provides a well-defined starting point for the activation of principal cells after each onset signal from the onset neurons. Since they are at the same time released from inhibition by tuberculoventral cells, the principal cells are able to then start with the summation of their input from the auditory nerve.

Direct evidence for such a summation process requires intracellular recording from principal cells in response to appropriate stimulation. Fig. 7.11 shows a preliminary result from a slice preparation of the gerbil CN; it indicates how a principal cell can summarize its input activity (Ochse, 1999). The responses of the cell were elicited with short current impulses to the membrane of the cell.

Obviously, principal cells may integrate a certain number of small current pulses before they generate a spike. Under the stimulus conditions in this case, the cell needed ten stimulus pulses (see inset of Fig. 7.11). One can only guess how many postsynaptic impulses from the auditory nerve would be needed to drive the cell, but it would certainly always be approximately the same provided the input pulses stay the same.

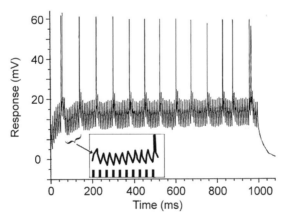

Fig. 7.11   The depicted intracellular recording from a principal cell is from a slice of the gerbil DCN. The cell was stimulated with tiny current pulses (1.2 nA, 3 ms duration, 8 ms period). The cell membrane potential increases slightly after each current pulse, especially at the beginning of the stimulation (see also membrane potential and stimulation pulses in the inset enlargement). Under the given stimulus conditions it takes ten current pulses for the membrane potential to reach its threshold and the cell to generate a spike (or two). Capacity effects conceal the integration process in later phases of the recording, but the nearly constant numbers of stimulation pulses that are necessary to elicit a spike indicate that the potential steps at the actual spike generation zone must be always the same (Ochse, 1999).

This would be the case for a periodic signal and, when the acoustic stimulus is coded by phase coupling, it should always be the same number of waves of the signal fine structure which elicit a spike in a principal cell.

Because of their size, the large principal cells (giant cells) have a large capacity. Consequently, they should have long time constants (25–40 ms) that make them appropriate for the coding of low frequencies or modulation frequencies. In contrast, the smaller principal cells (fusiform cells) are faster and more adapted to process higher frequencies. In order to code periodicity information over a wide range of frequencies, fusiform cells should provide a range of time constants for each possible carrier (or formant) frequency. Thus, a corresponding systematic array of fusiform cells with different time constants would be required along the isofrequency lines of the DCN.

Finally, inputs to the DCN from various other sources are transferred by the granule cells (see Fig. 7.10). For example, a feedback from the inferior colliculus may serve to enhance responses to a modulation in a particular frequency range and suppress responses to other modulations. This should support our capability to detect a sound source in a noisy environment. Other inputs to the granule cells allow, for example, somatosensory information from our vocal system to interfere with the periodicity processing in the DCN (Shore and Zhou, 2006).

8   Periodicity coding in the midbrain

8.1   Coding of complex sounds

8.1.1   Processing of species-specific vocalizations

In the early 1970s, the customary silence of the green woods surrounding the Max-Planck Institute for Biophysical Chemistry in Göttingen-Nikolausberg was disturbed by harsh animal cries. The strange grating sounds emanated from a hutch on the roof of one of the ivory towers of this renowned institute. Underneath, seemingly oblivious to the cacophony overhead, scientists in Professor Otto Creutzfeldt's neurophysiology department were busy investigating how the brain perceives and analyses olfactory, somatosensory, visual and auditory information. The hutch that was the source of these unusual cries housed helmeted guinea fowl (Fig. 8.1), the subjects of neurophysiological research for a team of four young scientists, Vreni Maier, Henning Schiech, Rainer Koch and myself, who were fascinated by their vocalizations.

We selected these long-necked relatives of pheasants for our research because we wanted to investigate the processing of species-specific vocalizations in their central auditory system. Our working hypothesis was that recognition of complex communication sounds might involve feature detectors, i.e. neurons which respond preferentially, if not exclusively, to particular combinations of acoustic parameters characteristic for these sounds.

As our investigations revealed (Maier, 1982; Scheich *et al.*, 1983), besides formants comparable to those in human vowels, another important feature of guinea fowl communication sounds is periodic amplitude modulation (AM) (Fig. 8.2). As harmony, formant structure and more or less rapid AMs are characteristic of many communication sounds, the neuronal coding of guinea fowl communication is an excellent model for auditory coding mechanisms in general, including human speech processing.

For our experiments we selected the auditory midbrain nucleus MLD (mesencephalicus lateralis, pars dorsalis), which in birds corresponds to the mammalian inferior colliculus. Our aim was to record from single neurons in the midbrain while the birds were sitting in a soundproof booth, listening to a tape recording of species-specific vocalizations.

Fig. 8.2a shows the results of such an experiment. A peri-stimulus time histogram (PSTH) summarizes the responses from a midbrain neuron in a hen with a strong

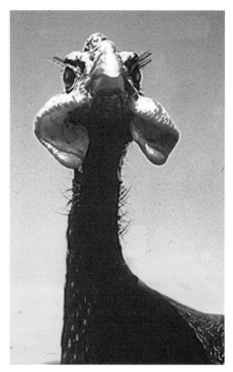

Fig. 8.1   A guinea cock, recognizable by his large (in reality red) lobes.

preference for an AM call from a guinea cock (Fig. 8.2b, c). The recording is a typical example of the faithful temporal representation of natural sounds in the auditory midbrain of birds (Scheich *et al.*, 1977). Both the rapid modulations around 40 Hz in the first part and the slow modulations between 6 and 8 Hz in the second part of the vocalization are apparent. Moreover, it turned out that at least in the midbrain of birds signal modulations, sometimes even up to 800 Hz, are represented with high fidelity (Fig. 8.3).

Quite rapid AMs characterize one of the vocalizations of guinea hens which – because of its characteristic rhythm – we called 'iambus'. It is based on a harmonic sound with a fundamental frequency of about 1000 Hz, while its modulation frequency varies around 330 Hz (period = 3 ms; Fig. 8.4a). This frequency combination often creates strong inharmonic sidebands that frame each of the harmonic components and are responsible for their rough timbre. Our behavioural observations showed that even after months of separation hens who utter such calls are recognized by their group individually and obtain feedback from their cocks (Maier, 1982).

Furthermore, our investigations showed that certain neurons in the midbrain do indeed prefer the iambus call over other sometimes remarkably similar sounds (Fig. 8.4b; Scheich *et al.*, 1983). These neurons were to a certain extent selective to carrier frequencies around 1000 Hz, or a harmonic thereof, provided it was modulated by a frequency of about 330 Hz.

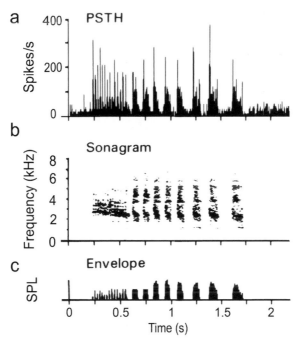

Fig. 8.2   (a) The PSTH (binwidth 5 ms) shows the temporal response of a neuron in the auditory midbrain of a guinea hen exposed to a species-specific vocalization (agitation call by a guinea cock; 20 repetitions, 65 dB SPL). The spectral analysis **(b)** and the fast and slow AMs of the signal envelope **(c)** are shown along the same time axis (modified from Scheich *et al.*, 1977).

We later found an even higher specificity to various natural calls in the guinea fowl forebrain (cortex analogue), especially highly selective responses to warning calls (Bonke *et al.*, 1979). This vocalization is a strange vibrating sound which is characterized by periodic amplitude and frequency modulations of a carrier frequency at about 2500 Hz (period = 0.4 ms! See Section 5.6) by a modulation frequency of 110 Hz.

8.1.2   Neuronal mechanisms of feature detection

It was particularly challenging to understand the neuronal mechanisms behind this type of feature detection. How are neurons in the auditory midbrain of the guinea fowl able to detect the presence of such modulated sounds and signal this to higher brain centres? Many neurons were obviously involved in processing AMs of around 110 Hz and 330 Hz, the two major modulation ranges of guinea fowl vocalizations, but in spite of this we had to conclude that these neurons did not care whether such modulations were actually part of a natural call or were artificially produced. A major function of the auditory midbrain was apparently the processing of amplitude modulations covering a great range of carrier and modulation frequencies. As it turned out, single neurons in the midbrain of guinea fowl, as well as of other species,

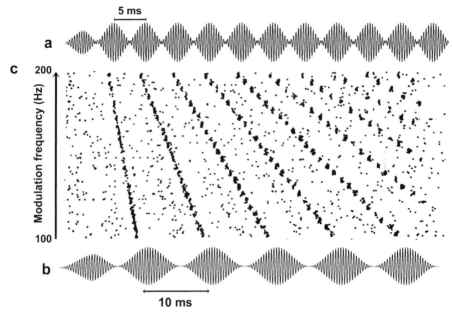

Fig. 8.3   Responses of a neuron in the auditory midbrain of a guinea hen synchronized to AMs.
(a) Scheme of an AM stimulus with a modulation frequency of 200 Hz (5 ms period; carrier
frequency: 2500 Hz: intensity ramp of 5 ms at the start; presented at 65 dB SPL). (b) The
same but with a modulation frequency of 100 Hz (10 ms period). (c) 'Point plot' (each
spike indicated as a dot) of the highly synchronized responses of the neuron to 100 repetitions
of 24 AM stimuli, as described above, with the modulation frequency changing from 200 Hz to
100 Hz in equal periodicity steps.

clearly respond very well to pure tones with a certain frequency, their characteristic
frequency (CF). But they usually respond much better when the amplitude of this
tone is modulated with a certain modulation frequency, their 'best modulation frequency' (BMF).

There was no doubt that the auditory analysis of complex signals must involve
more than the neuronal analysis of spectral information derived in the cochlea
and represented in tonotopic frequency maps in the central nervous system. At
the time we were investigating the coding of natural calls in guinea fowl (Scheich
et al., 1977), such considerations led others to conduct similar experiments
using natural sounds or AMs as stimuli (Møller, 1971; Suga and Schlegel, 1972;
Winter and Funkenstein, 1973; Bibikov, 1974; Moore and Cashin, 1974; Aertsen and
Johannesma, 1980).

The generally accepted conclusion from these investigations was that the selectivity
for particular signal properties increases as one ascends the hierarchy of the auditory
system. Neurons in the central auditory system are selective for a certain frequency
because they are connected directly or indirectly to a certain place on the basilar
membrane. In contrast, their possible selectivity for more complex features, such as a
modulation frequency, must result from complex connections and interactions with
other neurons in the brainstem and from their intrinsic temporal properties.

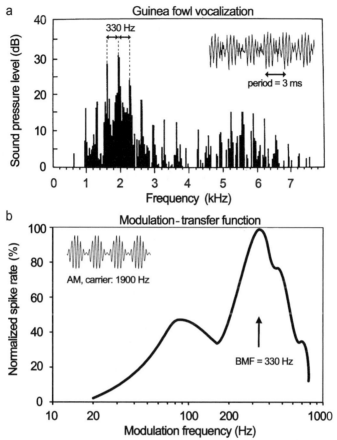

Fig. 8.4   **(a)** Spectrogram and oscillogram of a typical iambus call of a guinea hen. The carrier of the AM vocalization is a harmonic sound with a fundamental of about 970 Hz; due to the AM (see inset) each harmonic is accompanied by a lower and an upper sideband at a distance of about 330 Hz, well visible above and below 1940 Hz (second harmonic; see arrows). **(b)** Modulation-transfer function (MTF; see Box 7.1) of a neuron in the midbrain of a guinea fowl with a preference for a modulation around 330 Hz and a carrier frequency of 1900 Hz.

8.2   Synchronization and rate

A high percentage of neurons in the midbrain prefer a certain modulation frequency, recognizable either by their maximal synchronization to corresponding signals (see Box 8.1) or by their maximal average activity. As an example, Fig. 8.5b shows the MTFs of a neuron recorded in the auditory midbrain of a guinea hen. This neuron synchronized to modulation frequencies between about 50 and 250 Hz, but preferred to fire with a maximal spike rate at a modulation frequency (its rate-BMF) of 160 Hz.

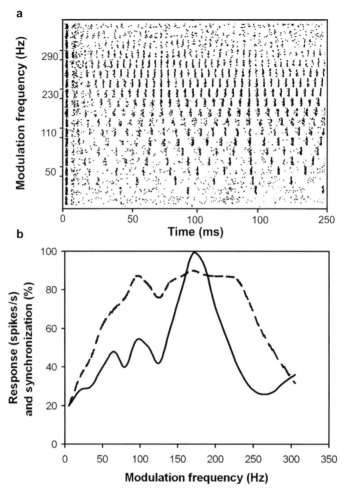

Fig. 8.5   (a) 'Point plot' of a neuronal response in the auditory midbrain of a guinea hen to 19 modulation frequencies varied in equal periodicity steps from 5 Hz to 235 Hz (carrier frequency: 1800 Hz; intensity: 65 dB SPL; 30 repetitions). (b) MTFs measured by average response (solid line) and synchronization (vector strength; dashed line). The neuron is highly synchronized over more than two octaves of modulation frequencies, but narrowly tuned in terms of response rate to its BMF of 160 Hz.

It is a common finding that neuronal synchronization to higher modulation frequencies deteriorates at increasingly higher levels of the auditory system. While in the auditory nerve even modulations above 5000 Hz are encoded to a certain extent (see Fig. 7.1), at the level of the midbrain the temporal acuity of responses to modulations above 300 Hz tends to be significantly diminished. This was demonstrated in a variety of species (Rees and Møller, 1983; Langner, 1992; Bodnar and Bass, 2001; Langner *et al.*, 2002; Rees and Langner, 2005). Alternatively, neurons signal periodicity information to higher processing centres by means of their spike rate and their spatial position in the midbrain. This type of coding is called 'labelled line' or 'rate-place' coding.

BOX 8.1   Measures of synchronization

A simple way to visualize synchronized responses of a neuron is by means of a so-called period histogram. These diagrams show how neuronal spikes are distributed on average over a stimulus period.

Quantitatively, the synchronization may be evaluated by the use of circular statistics (Langner, 1992; Rees and Langner, 2005). If the period of a signal is represented by a circle, a spike appearing at a certain time during a period of the signal may be represented by a vector $\vec{a_i}$ with unit length. The direction of the vector indicates the phase angle in which the spike appears during a period.

Fig. 8.1.1 shows the sum of two vectors $\vec{a_i}$ and $\vec{a_2}$ (left) which represent two spikes a_1 and a_2 (right) of a neuronal response during two subsequent periods of a sine wave.

The vector sum $\vec{R} = \sum_{i=1}^{N} \vec{a_i}$ over all N spike vectors of a response characterizes the neuronal synchronization. The length of the vector $\vec{R}$ is a measure of the total synchronized response and its direction indicates the corresponding mean phase angle. Finally, the 'vector strength' is a measure for the average degree of response synchronization and may be obtained by dividing the vector sum by the number N of the involved spikes $\vec{r} = \vec{R}/N$.

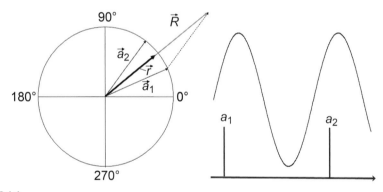

Fig. 8.1.1

In spite of the general decrease of temporal coding, some neurons in the midbrain synchronize to low modulation frequencies as well as, or sometimes even better than, auditory nerve fibres (Figs. 8.5, 8.6; Rose and Capranica, 1985; Epping and Eggermont, 1986). Moreover, synchronization to still quite high modulation frequencies has been demonstrated in the midbrain of different animals: in cats up to 600 Hz (Fig. 8.6c; Langner and Schreiner, 1988), in bats up to 800 Hz (Lesser *et al.*, 1986) and in guinea fowl up to 1000 Hz (Langner, 1981, 1983).

The periodicity range between about 30 and 1000 Hz is the most relevant for human voices and consequently also for pitch in speech and music. This range of periodicity

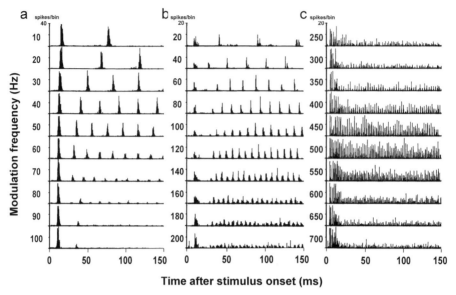

Fig. 8.6   PSTHs of synchronized responses of three neurons in the midbrain of a cat to periodic amplitude
modulations (100% modulation depths; ten different modulation frequencies as indicated at the
left). The characteristic frequencies (CFs) of the neurons were chosen as carrier frequencies
(a: 21.5 kHz, b: 11.5 kHz; c: 3.1 kHz). The signal intensities were 30 dB above the thresholds of
the neurons. The scaling of the PSTHs is 40 **(a)** and 20 **(b, c)** spikes per bin (binwidth 0.04 ms;
modified from Langner and Schreiner, 1988).

covers nearly five of the seven octaves that are represented, for example, on a piano.
The same range is also covered by the distributions of BMFs of neurons in the
midbrain (inferior colliculus) of the cat (Fig. 8.7) and of various other animals
(Langner and Schreiner, 1988; Langner *et al.*, 2002; Rees and Langner, 2005). In
line with the idea of a transformation into a rate-place code, the rate-related distributions are broad and extend up to 1000 Hz (Fig. 8.8a,c,e,f), while the synchronization-
based distributions (Fig. 8.8b,d) give a further indication of a reduction of temporal
coding above about 150 Hz.

8.3   Stimulus parameters and response features

A minority of periodicity coding neurons in the midbrain were found to be quite
sensitive to various parameter changes. For example, changing the signal intensity
may change the shape, including the peak position, of their MTFs (Rees and Palmer,
1989; Krishna and Semple, 2000). Sometimes, even the low-pass characteristics that
neurons exhibit at low sound intensities may change into band pass at higher levels
(Rees and Møller, 1987).

In contrast, for the majority of investigated midbrain neurons periodicity tuning
turned out to be quite robust against variations of various signal parameters.

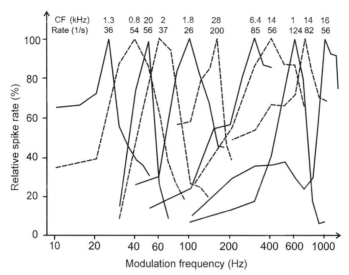

Fig. 8.7 In contrast to more peripheral auditory nuclei, many neurons in the midbrain have MTFs with band-pass properties. The figure shows sharply tuned MTFs that cover the most relevant periodicity range below 1000 Hz. Numbers above the curves indicate the CF (carrier frequency of the AM stimuli) and the maximal firing rate of the neurons (modified from Langner and Schreiner, 1988).

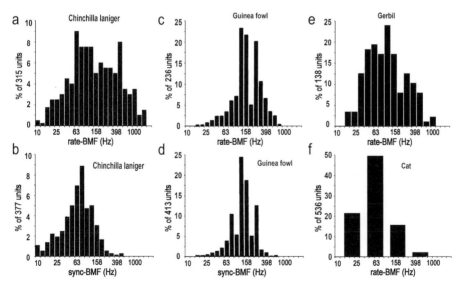

Fig. 8.8 The distributions of modulation tuning in the auditory midbrain of different animals are based on the measurement of either response rates **(a, c, e, f)** or synchronization **(b, d)**. Especially in the chinchilla **(a)** and gerbil **(e)** the rate-based distributions are broad, extending up to 1000 Hz, while the synchronization-based distributions **(b, d)** indicate a reduction of temporal coding above about 150 Hz. Although experimental conditions have to be taken into account, the distributions in **(c)** and **(d)** suggest that there may be a predominance of neurons devoted to the processing of species-specific vocalizations in the midbrain of the guinea fowl (compare Fig. 8.4).

In addition, many neurons were found to be consistently synchronized to the envelope of AM signals over a wide range of stimulus levels and modulation depths (Brugge *et al.*, 1993; Zschau, 2008). In various animals, including frogs and bats, neurons may synchronize to AM signals modulated by only 2% (Schuller, 1979; Rees and Møller, 1983; Bibikov and Nizamov, 1996). In bats, this neuronal coding feature certainly contributes to their amazing ability to distinguish mealworms from less delicious food 'simply' by their ultrasonic echoes.

A major parameter of an AM signal is its carrier frequency. We know from Chapter 4 that the shift of the carrier frequency results in a shift of the pitch of an AM signal (pitch-shift effect). Accordingly, the variation of this parameter also has a strong influence on the MTFs of the midbrain neurons (see Section 9.5). Even small changes to the carrier frequency of AM signals often result in a significant increase or decrease of the BMF of a neuron (Langner, 1983; Langner and Schreiner, 1988; Krishna and Semple, 2000). This detuning of periodicity coding neurons may offer an explanation of the pitch-shift effect. Finally, since periodicity pitch can be perceived by various animals (cat: Chung and Colavita, 1976; Heffner and Whitfield, 1976; bird: Cynx and Shapiro, 1986; monkey: Schwarz and Tomlinson, 1990), and the BMF-shift effect was also demonstrated in the midbrain of a variety of animal species including the frog (Walkowiak, 1984), one would expect that behavioural experiments might also reveal the pitch-shift effect in animals.

8.4   Periodicity coding

8.4.1   Temporal response patterns

As we have seen above, many neurons in the midbrain respond preferentially to particular modulation frequencies, some with more or less precise synchronization, but most of them with an increase in their average spike rate. The particular way a neuron codes periodicity is the result of specific temporal properties which to a large degree reflect the complex interactions of their input neurons.

Many midbrain neurons show more than just an increase in their average spike activity, and the details of their temporal response patterns make it possible to infer the underlying coding mechanisms. As an example, a point plot histogram is shown in Fig. 8.9a for such a neuron in the guinea fowl midbrain. The neuron was investigated using ten different modulation frequencies between 100 and 1000 Hz (equidistant periods: 10 to 1 ms); the carrier of the AM signal at 2 kHz was at the CF of the neuron. The BMF both for synchronization and for rate was about 330 Hz (3 ms period). A simplified and feature-enhanced version of this 'point plot' (Fig. 8.9b) is used to demonstrate five temporal response properties which are relevant for periodicity coding in general. These five properties are:

(1) *Intrinsic oscillations*: perhaps the most noticeable response feature is the intrinsic oscillations which are triggered with a short latency at each signal onset and at each

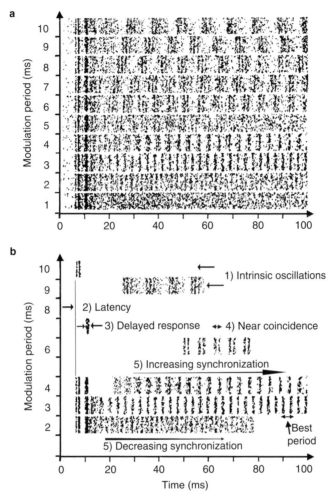

Fig. 8.9 (a) The diagram shows responses of a neuron in the midbrain of a guinea fowl to ten different AM signals (carrier frequency: 2 kHz, modulation depth: 100%, level: 65 dB SPL; 100 repetitions; spikes plotted as points along the time axis in a separate array for each modulation frequency). The best modulation period for synchronization and rate is about 3 ms (~330 Hz modulation frequency). (b) The simplified version of the same diagram brings out the temporal response properties of the neuron: (1) intrinsic oscillations which are triggered with a short latency at each signal onset and modulation cycle; (2) the onset latency; (3) a slightly stronger delayed response clearly discernible at each onset; (4) a near coincidence of the delayed and oscillatory components; (5) increasing and decreasing synchronization below and above the best modulation period.

modulation cycle. At the onset, the neuron shown in Fig. 8.9 oscillates with a period of about 1.2 ms (the period increases slightly in the responses to the individual modulation cycles).

(2) *Onset latency*: the onset or response latency of a neuron is usually determined by stimulation with a pure tone at its CF. It is readily understandable that it takes a few

milliseconds until the neuron starts to respond to such a stimulus. Most of the latency is due to the time it takes for the neuronal signal to reach the midbrain (~4–5 ms in guinea fowl). The observed latency is slightly longer than this because, as we will see below, it is prolonged by one period of the intrinsic oscillation. This additional delay can be explained by two assumptions: first, the intrinsic oscillation is already contained in the input to this neuron, and second, the corresponding input neuron, presumably a chopper neuron in the CN, needs one oscillation period to produce its first spike. This delay component, due to intrinsic oscillations, seems to contribute to the latency of all periodicity-tuned neurons in the midbrain (see also Figs. 8.13a, 8.14).

(3) *Delayed non-oscillatory response*: while the intrinsic oscillation fades away within a few milliseconds of onset (before it is triggered again by the subsequent modulation cycles), a slightly stronger non-oscillatory response is clearly discernible about 11 ms after each signal onset. Like the oscillations, these delayed spikes are a temporal feature of many periodicity-tuned neurons. The interval between the first onset spikes and the delayed response approximates the period of the BMF – in this case about 3.2 ms. In the next chapter I will present a periodicity model which may explain this relationship.

(4) *Near coincidence of delayed and oscillatory components*: the delayed responses are triggered not only by the signal onset but also, just like the intrinsic oscillations, by each cycle of the amplitude modulation. However, they are separable from the oscillatory responses only under certain favourable temporal conditions that are provided by the appropriate modulation frequencies. As a result, a near coincidence of the delayed and 'relatively undelayed' oscillatory response components arises. Both components only coincide sufficiently to elicit a strong combined response at the BMF.

(5) *Synchronization increase and decrease*: the neuron only shows a strong synchronized response to all modulation cycles at the best modulation period (~3 ms). Above this modulation period the synchronization increases, below this period it decreases over time. This implies (and can be seen in the responses) that the coincidence of the delayed with the oscillatory input is improving over time for the higher and deteriorating for the lower modulation period. This is another temporal effect which can be observed in the responses of many midbrain neurons and for which the periodicity model presented in the next chapter will provide an explanation.

8.4.2   Coincidence effect

While the coincidence of inputs with different delays cannot be directly seen in Fig. 8.9, it is visible in the responses of other periodicity-tuned neurons. An example of such a neuron from the midbrain of a guinea fowl is shown in Fig. 8.10. In this case, 30 different modulation frequencies were imposed on carrier frequencies of 2.8 kHz (a) and 3 kHz (b). In both of the point plots,

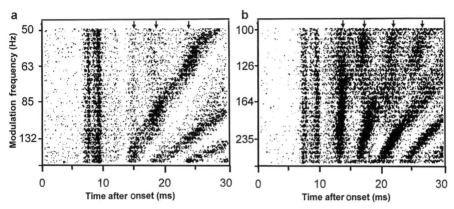

Fig. 8.10   The 'point plots' bring out the coincidence effect. They show responses of a neuron in the midbrain of a guinea hen to 30 AM signals (carrier frequencies: **(a)** 2.8 kHz; **(b)** 3 kHz; modulation depth: 100%; level: 65 dB SPL; 100 repetitions; spikes plotted in a separate array for each modulation frequency). In both diagrams arrows point to delayed responses to the onset and to the subsequent modulation cycles. Where delayed inputs coincide with (nearly) undelayed inputs to the later cycles (resulting in sloping bands of activity) strong responses are elicited (dark point clusters below the arrows). The coincidence effect explains the preferences of the recorded neuron for modulation frequencies of about 100 Hz **(a)** and 235 Hz **(b)**.

arrows mark vertical clusters of points which arise from responses to delayed inputs (i.e. with a relatively large delay) that are synchronized to the onset of the signal. In contrast, the sloping clusters originate from responses to inputs that synchronize (with much less delay) to the subsequent modulation cycles. The highest density of points results from the coincidence of the inputs that respond with a delay to the onset (vertical point clouds) with the much less delayed input responses (sloping point clouds) to the following modulation cycles. (Note that 100 repetitions of the stimulus make it possible to see the responses to inputs even without coincidences.)

The conclusion from these response patterns is that a coincidence neuron can elicit a strong response when the period of the stimulus modulation just matches the delay differences of its inputs. It is only in this case that the delayed response – to earlier signal parts – can add (or multiply) with the (nearly) undelayed responses to later parts of the signal.

8.5   Intrinsic oscillations

Many neurons in the midbrain of experimental animals show intrinsic oscillations, short bursts of spikes synchronized either to the onsets of tones or to individual modulation cycles of AM sounds (Figs. 8.9, 8.11). It is not surprising that these responses so closely resemble those of the chopper cells in the CN. As we now know, these neurons provide

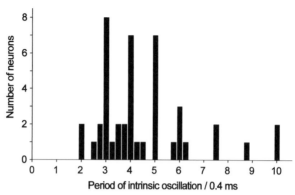

Fig. 8.11   Many neurons in the midbrain show distinct intrinsic oscillations with preferences for oscillation periods which are multiples of a base period of 0.4 ms. In the given example from the cat the distribution shows peaks at intervals of 1.2, 1.6, 2.0 and 2.4 ms (only the first period of each oscillation after stimulus onset was considered; from Langner and Schreiner, 1988).

the dominant input to the midbrain (Adams, 1983) and hence must have a major influence on responses in the midbrain.

Our early experiments in guinea fowl, and later in various other animals, made it increasingly clear that the periods of these oscillations were not equally distributed. Instead, there seemed to be a rather puzzling preference for periods that were small integer multiples of a base period of 0.4 ms (Langner, 1983). As we have seen in Chapters 4 and 5, the constant of 0.4 ms should be considered as a kind of universal auditory time constant that shows up not only in pitch perception (Langner, 1981, 1985), but also in related but quite different fields of hearing and sound production.

When Christoph Schreiner from the University of California in San Francisco and I were investigating periodicity coding in the midbrain of the cat (Langner and Schreiner, 1988), we found evidence for the same time constant in intrinsic oscillations in this animal. Moreover, we were able to demonstrate that the oscillation periods were only weakly influenced by changes in intensity or stimulus frequency (Fig. 8.12). This would be expected if the oscillations are elicited by inputs from chopper neurons in the CN which are also characterized by interspike intervals that are largely unrelated to these stimulus parameters (see Section 7.2.5; Pfeiffer, 1966).

If the assumption that intrinsic oscillations in the midbrain simply echo those of chopper neurons in the CN is right, the preferred intervals should also be a feature of these midbrain neurons. We found some direct evidence for this hypothesis in a paper analysing the temporal properties of neurons in the CN of the cat, published in 1988 by Eric Young and co-workers from the Johns Hopkins University School of Medicine, Baltimore (Young *et al.*, 1988). When we analysed their data regarding the preference for certain chopper intervals, it turned out that their recorded 'regular chopper neurons' do indeed show a significant preference for oscillation intervals centred at multiples of

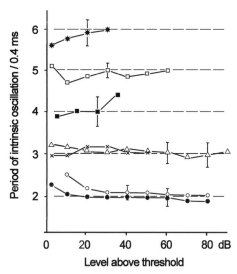

Fig. 8.12 The intensity dependence of intrinsic oscillations of seven neurons in the midbrain of the cat. Stimulation of the neurons at different levels above their response threshold at CF elicited short oscillatory responses. At higher levels the mean interspike intervals approached different integer multiples of 0.4 ms (modified from Langner and Schreiner, 1988).

0.4 ms (Bahmer and Langner, 2006a). While this finding provides a reasonable explanation for the existence of intrinsic oscillations in the midbrain and their temporal features, it leaves open the question of how the properties of chopper neurons can be explained in the first place. This is one of the questions that will be addressed in the next chapter (see Section 9.4).

8.6 Best modulation period, intrinsic oscillation and onset latency

A neuron in the midbrain may be characterized by three temporal parameters: the period of its BMF and the period of its intrinsic oscillation and its (response or onset) latency. A statistical evaluation of the response properties of 250 neurons in the midbrain of the cat showed how these parameters are related (Fig. 8.13). On average, the latency is prolonged by one period of an intrinsic oscillation (latency = 7 ms + τ_{osci}) as indicated by the fitted line in Fig. 8.13a. This relation may be explained by the assumption that the neuron is driven by an oscillatory input of which the first spike comes only after the first oscillation period (see also Section 8.4.2).

The plot in Fig. 8.13b shows the corresponding statistical relationship between the periods of the BMF (τ_{BMF}) of the neurons and their intrinsic oscillation. As it turns out, τ_{BMF} of the neurons is on average equal to six periods of their oscillation period ($\tau_{BMF} = 6 \cdot \tau_{osci}$; $\tau_{osci} = \tau_{BMF}/6$). The size of the error bars indicates that this is a good fit for most but not all neurons.

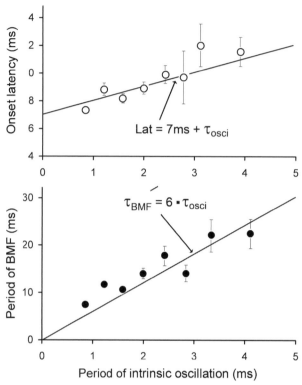

Fig. 8.13 (a) The mean periods of intrinsic oscillations (τ_{osci}) of 250 neurons in the midbrain of the cat was correlated (a) with their onset latency (Lat) and (b) with the period of their BMF (τ_{BMF}). The matching lines show theoretical predictions – as indicated. The bars designate standard deviations of the distributions. Extremely long latencies were ignored (Nalimov outlier test, $p = 95\%$).

Together these data support the conclusions that we had already reached from an analysis of recordings from over 600 neurons in the cat midbrain (Langner *et al.*, 1987b; Fig. 8.14). Clearly, the average response latency of the recorded neurons strongly depends on their best modulation frequency. We have already seen that this is due to the contribution of oscillatory components to the latency. However, there are also other parameters that influence the latency as measured in such experiments. These include not only a constant neuronal delay from the cochlea to the midbrain, but also the delay as the sound travels from the sound transmitter through the outer and middle ear to the cochlea, as well as the travel time of the waves on the basilar membrane. The time needed by the wave to reach its point of maximal deflection is slightly larger than one period of the stimulating frequency. Therefore, a delay of this size is also included in the latency of neurons tuned to this frequency (Ruggero and Rich, 1987). Thus, in the cat the relationship between the latency, the constant delay to

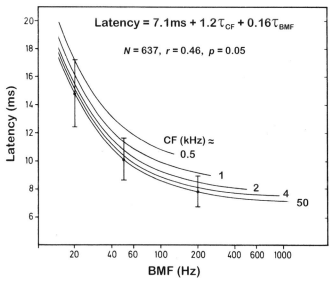

Fig. 8.14　On average, the response latency of neurons in the midbrain of the cat depends strongly on their BMF. The shift of the different curves shows the effect of the CF. Due to the delay introduced by the travelling wave in the cochlea, neurons with a lower CF have a slightly longer latency than neurons with a higher CF (modified from Langner *et al.*, 1987b).

the midbrain (7.1 ms), the CF and the BMF of the neurons can be summarized by a simple equation (Langner *et al.*, 1987b):

$$\text{Lat} = 7.1 \text{ ms} + 1.2 \cdot \tau_{CF} + \tau_{BMF}/6$$

Since for most neurons even about one-sixth of the period of a BMF is larger than the delay introduced by the travelling wave ($\sim$1/CF), the latency variation across the population of periodicity-tuned midbrain neurons is mainly due to this parameter (τ_{BMF}).

9 Theories of periodicity coding

9.1 Synchronization and harmony

In early 1976 I was standing chest-deep in the water of a flooded island, not far from the mouth of the Rio Negro, whose black water could still be seen alongside the white floods of the Amazon. The reason for this (for me, at least) unusual location was that my colleagues and I, accompanied by experts and fishermen from the Instituto Nacional de Pesquisas da Amazônia in Manaus, were fishing with nets and had to remove the water plants in which our prey – various species of electric fish – was hiding.

These fish are able to orientate and communicate in this dull environment using only their weak electric signals, and we wanted to study the amazing neuronal networks that make this possible. The result was worth all the trouble. One of the things we discovered later in the laboratory was that a certain electric fish (*Sternarchorhamphus*), which generates electrical signals with frequencies well above 1000 Hz, was able to couple its sinusoidal signals in phase with our electronic generators (Fig. 9.1; Langner and Scheich, 1978).

Another observation was that their phase-coupling could be one to one, but could also be in other harmonic relationships. This finding was in line with the near octave (1:2) relationship of the signals from males and females of another electric fish, *Sternopygus macrurus*, which was observed during courtship behaviour (Hopkins, 1974). Since our own haul produced a variety of species of electric fish that use different frequencies, we were able to see that *Sternarchorhynchus* also phase-coupled to signals of other species. Some of these discharged signals were several hundred Hertz below their own frequency and for a short time the two frequencies would stay in a harmonic relation, e.g. 2:3, 2:5 or 1:3 (mosquitoes use – for the same purpose – their wing-beat frequency; Warren *et al.*, 2009; Gibson *et al.*, 2010). One may only speculate to what ends these fish have developed these amazing capabilities, but at that time it convinced me that synchronization and harmony are options of neuronal systems in general and that neurons must be able to temporally analyse quite high frequencies with microsecond precision.

9.2 The Licklider model

Theories that our central hearing system is able to deal with high frequencies and to perform some kind of a temporal analysis, like a neuronal correlation, have been around

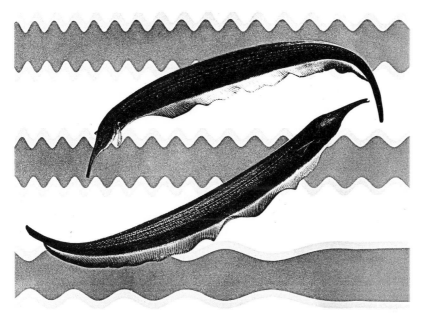

Fig. 9.1   Many species of electric fish, for example in the Amazon River, use near-sinusoidal weak electric signals to explore their environment and to communicate with each other. Individuals of *Sternarchorhamphus* use frequencies as high as 1500 Hz. The pattern of decelerating beats shown in the background of the picture demonstrates that these fishes, in contrast to other species which prefer their own frequencies, occasionally couple their signal in phase with those of other individuals (from Langner and Scheich, 1978).

for many years (see Box 9.1). The one that is best known was advanced in 1951 by J. C. R. Licklider (Fig. 9.2). He postulated that the quasi-Fourier analysis in the cochlea is followed by a correlation analysis in the cochlear nucleus (CN). In his famous 'Duplex-theory' paper (Licklider, 1951), he pointed out:

The stimulus basis for pitch is duplex: On the one hand we have frequency, on the other hand, periodicity. That frequency and period are reciprocally related is not sufficient reason for throwing one away and examining only the other, for with each one is associated a method of analysis. Of the two methods, one – frequency analysis performed by an array of band pass filters – has been incorporated into auditory theory. The cochlea is almost universally regarded as being an extended wave filter that distributes oscillations of different frequencies to different places. The possibility that the other method, autocorrelational analysis, plays a role in the auditory process has been neglected.

To a certain extent this last statement still holds, even 60 years later. According to Licklider, a correlation analysis is carried out entirely within the time domain but yields the same information as the power spectrum obtained through analysis in the frequency domain. The inventor of cybernetics, Norbert Wiener, showed that these functions are simply related by a Fourier transformation. Licklider realized that the attractiveness of the correlation analysis lies in the fact that the necessary mechanisms

BOX 9.1 Correlation analysis

Fig. 9.1.1 demonstrates the general principle of a correlation analysis, a powerful mathematical method used to analyse the periodicity of a signal in the time domain.

(a) A sonagram of a human vowel. The dark areas indicate high amplitudes of formants and vertical stripes indicate modulations due to the fundamental frequency of the vowel.
(b) The same only simplified.
(c) A 'party effect': a superposed vowel with different formants and fundamental makes it difficult to recognize vowel formants and identity.
(d) The periodicity of the signal in (a) and (b) is extracted and a corresponding signal with an arbitrary delay is superposed over the mixed signals in (c): the resulting beat pattern makes it easy to separate the two.

Similarly, in order to analyse a periodic signal in the brain, delayed and undelayed neuronal responses to the signal envelope are required which then converge on neurons functioning as coincidence detectors. The autocorrelation analysis ('auto' indicates that a signal is compared with itself) is the corresponding mathematical formalism, where the amplitudes of a delayed and an undelayed version of a signal are multiplied 'point by point' and the result is summed up (see Box 9.2).

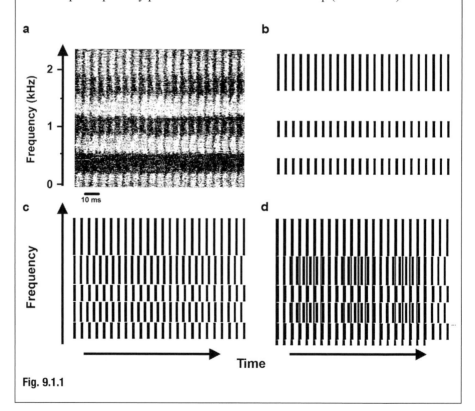

Fig. 9.1.1

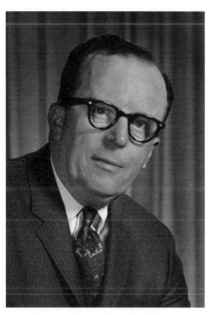

Fig. 9.2   Joseph Carl Robnett Licklider (1915–1990) started his career as a psychologist. His doctoral thesis (Licklider, 1941) was concerned with tonotopy in the auditory cortex of the cat. In the following years, as a research fellow at Harvard University, he advanced theories of pitch perception and the intelligibility of speech. He was also a recognized computer pioneer – his 'Galactic Network' concept, proposed in 1962, was very similar to the internet of today (www.thocp.net/biographies/licklidder_jcr.html).

are quite different from those involved in the frequency analysis. While the frequency analysis is performed by the cochlea, the correlation takes place in the central nervous system.

According to Licklider, the auditory system is well set up to perform a 'running correlation analysis' (Fig. 9.3). The cochlea performs a 'crude frequency analysis by distributing different frequency bands to different positions', i.e. to different hair cells and nerve fibres along the basilar membrane. The spikes elicited by neuron A are carried by the auditory nerve to many autocorrelators working in parallel. Via a chain of neurons (B), each autocorrelator provides a delay axis orthogonal to the frequency axis. The necessary multiplication of delayed and undelayed inputs is executed by coincidence neurons (C). Finally, the resulting responses are integrated over a certain time period by the integration neurons (D).

Licklider presented his model more than half a century ago, however, and some of his assumptions have since turned out to be unrealistic. First of all, the delay chains that are required for his model are present neither in the CN nor anywhere else in the brain. Also, as a single synaptic delay is so short (<1 ms), the chains of neurons would have to be extremely long to account for the coding of low pitches (in order to produce, for example, a 50 ms delay). At the time it was not known that the CN

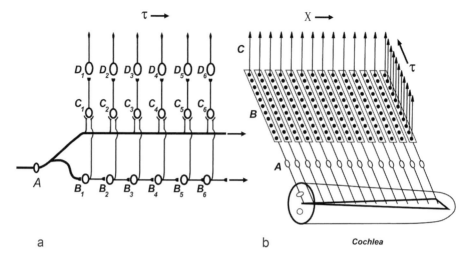

a   b   *Cochlea*

Fig. 9.3   **(a)** In Licklider's 'neuronal autocorrelator' the input signal from neuron A arrives at coincidence
neurons C_n via the neurons B_k in a chain with synaptic delays and via an undelayed axonal input.
When the input signal is periodic the delayed and the undelayed signals arrive simultaneously at a
particular neuron C_n, which will be activated provided the delay is equal to the period. The two
coinciding inputs are multiplied and then integrated over a certain time by the corresponding
neuron D_n. These operations correspond to the mathematical definition of a 'running
autocorrelation' function. The D_k neurons provide a display of this function with the temporal
course of discharges at A as the input function (Licklider, 1951). **(b)** Licklider's 'overall analyser'.
The uncoiled cochlea performs a 'crude frequency analysis distributing different frequency bands
to different positions' (X). The resulting signals are carried by the auditory nerve to
autocorrelators. Each autocorrelator provides a delay axis (τ) orthogonal to the x-axis and
functions as described in **(a)**. The activity in the (x, τ) plane provides a 'progressive analysis' of the
acoustic stimulus, 'first in frequency and then in periodicity' (Licklider, 1951).

contains neurons with particular response properties (onset, chopper and pauser)
which probably contribute to the correlation analysis (see Section 9.3) and can
substitute for the unrealistically long delay chains which Licklider postulated.
Consequently, the model could not account for certain effects such as the pitch-
shift effects (see Chapter 3) which, in contrast to Schouten's residue, are not
mentioned in Licklider's paper.

9.3   The model of Hewitt and Meddis

Many models of temporal analysis have been suggested over the years (Stokkum, 1987;
Stokkum and Gielen, 1989; Dau *et al.*, 1997; Large and Crawford, 2002; Schneider
et al., 2005; Eguia *et al.*, 2010; for a review, see de Cheveigné, 2005), but, in principle,
none of them showed as many similarities to the periodicity model suggested in this
chapter (see Fig. 9.5) as did the Duplex theory. This is somewhat surprising because, just
as with the periodicity model, some models were actually designed explicitly to explain
the modulation tuning that we had found in the midbrain.

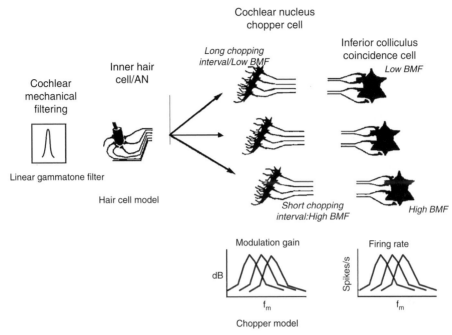

Cochlear nucleus
chopper cell

Inferior colliculus
coincidence cell

*Long chopping
interval/Low BMF*

Low BMF

Inner hair
cell/AN

Cochlear
mechanical
filtering

Linear gammatone filter

Hair cell model

*Short chopping
interval:High BMF*

High BMF

Modulation gain

dB

f_m

Firing rate

Spikes/s

f_m

Chopper model

Fig. 9.4   In contrast to the Licklider correlation model, in the Hewitt and Meddis model (above), the resonance properties of chopper neurons are crucial for periodicity tuning. The first two stages of the model (left side) represent cochlear filtering and inner hair cell transduction. The third stage (middle) includes the chopper neurons of the CN. A large number of identical chopper neurons synchronize best to the same modulation frequency. They converge on a single coincidence neuron in the midbrain (right side) which therefore responds with its highest spike rate to the BMF of its input neurons.

Perhaps the best example of such a model was suggested by Hewitt and Meddis (Fig. 9.4; Meddis and Hewitt, 1991; Hewitt *et al.*, 1992; Meddis and O'Mard, 1997); their model ascribes a major role to the intrinsic oscillations of chopper neurons. However, in contrast to the duplex theory and also the periodicity model (Fig. 9.5), the way the tuning of the coincidence neurons is achieved in the Hewitt and Meddis model is different – neuronal delays introduced, for example, by a chain of neurons (Fig. 9.3a) or by a temporal integration (Fig. 9.5b) do not play a role. Instead, the coincidence neurons are tuned to a particular modulation frequency (best modulation frequency – BMF) because each of them receives input from a large number of chopper neurons which are all tuned to the same BMF.

The attractiveness of the model of Hewitt and Meddis comes from the fact that it includes detailed modelling of the auditory periphery. In addition, the modulation-transfer functions of the simulated coincidence neurons are quite similar to those that we had actually observed in the midbrain (Langner and Schreiner, 1988). Simulation of the mechanical filtering and frequency selectivity of the cochlear was achieved by using the 'gammatone filter', which is quite popular among auditory modellers (Patterson *et al.*, 1986).

The simulation of chopper neurons revealed a number of properties characteristic of real chopper neurons, although it was necessary to assume an unrealistically high number of inputs from auditory nerve fibres (up to 60 instead of actually 3–5; see Fig. 7.10), all with the same characteristic frequency. The same problem arises at the stage of the coincidence neurons; a population of chopper neurons (up to 30) have to converge on a single coincidence neuron to achieve their typical modulation tuning. In the periodicity model the problem is mostly avoided by the function of the trigger neuron (Fig. 9.5).

The tuning of the coincidence neurons in the Hewitt and Meddis model reflects convergence of inputs from choppers with the same chopping frequency and, therefore, sensitivity to the same modulation frequency. As a result, the response rate of coincidence neurons is sensitive to the amplitude modulation and the maximal response is determined by the BMF of the input chopper neurons.

The fact that this model is able to simulate properties of coincidence neurons in the midbrain by relying on their input from chopper neurons indicates that these latter neurons must play an important role in the periodicity analysis. However, besides the unrealistically high convergence of inputs to chopper and coincidence neurons mentioned above, there are other drawbacks to the model. For instance, in order to code pitch for all relevant frequencies, the periods of intrinsic oscillations would have to be long enough to correspond to very low pitches (as low as 16 Hz). Such long periods are beyond the period range of up to about 8 ms which was observed in the CN of cats (Young *et al.*, 1988) as well as in the midbrain of various animals (Langner, 1992).

Moreover, the period of the intrinsic oscillation of a coincidence neuron in the midbrain was about one-sixth of the BMF period of a modulation-tuned neuron (see Fig. 8.13) while the model of Hewitt and Meddis predicts that these periods should always be equal. The model also cannot explain various details of temporal response patterns (see Figs. 6.13, 6.14) and, perhaps even more importantly, it is unable to explain the effect of pitch shifts or pitch steps (see Chapters 4 and 5). These inconsistencies indicate that, in spite of the fact that the model is relatively simple and able to make predictions, essential elements must be missing.

9.4   The periodicity model

9.4.1   The functional principle

Popular models, like those discussed above, do not explain essential known physiological and psychophysical aspects. However, one should never expect models to explain everything; rather, they should be as simple as possible but still explain, as precisely as possible, all of the really relevant aspects.

The periodicity model which is presented in this section (Fig. 9.5) was originally designed to explain the response properties of periodicity-tuned neurons in the midbrain. It is based on the observation that the input to the midbrain is temporally synchronized to the signal envelopes (but only broadly tuned in terms of rate;

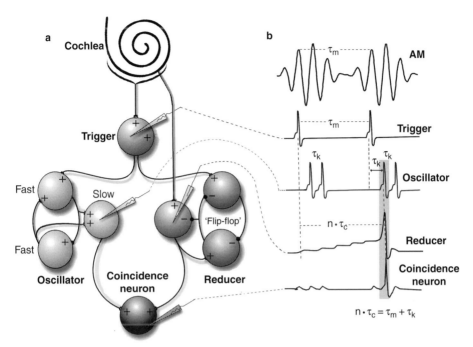

Fig. 9.5 (a) The neuronal periodicity circuit shown presents one of thousands of similar parallel circuits which together provide a complex network for a temporal correlation analysis. Each circuit combines four different neuronal components with features which can be attributed to real neurons or networks in the brainstem. The four components of the model are a trigger neuron, an oscillator and a reducer network with their neuronal counterparts in the CN and a coincidence neuron with its counterpart in the midbrain. (b) As indicated at the top, an amplitude-modulated (AM) signal is the assumed cochlear input. The way the model functions is illustrated by 'neuronal recordings'. Since the trigger neuron gets its input from a broad range of the cochlea (indicated by a bracket) it is able to synchronize to the envelope periods of the signal. It triggers oscillator and reducer responses that are consequently also synchronized to the signal. In order to reach the threshold, the main neuron of the reducer circuit (shown with an electrode) has to integrate a certain number (n) of spikes from the auditory nerve which are synchronized to the signal fine structure (e.g. the carrier of an AM signal). Therefore, the neuron responds after a certain phase delay (n · τ_c). In order to obtain a strong response from the coincidence neuron, the coincidence condition (n · $\tau_c = \tau_m + \tau_k$) has to be fulfilled: i.e. the phase delay of the reducer has to be compensated by the delay due to the periods of the signal (τ_m) and of the oscillation (τ_k).

see Figs. 7.7, 7.9). As will be discussed later (Chapter 11), the periodicity model can not only explain important aspects of pitch perception but also of harmony.

As Licklider has shown, a correlation analysis is a wonderful tool with which neurons can analyse periodicity information. For this purpose, delayed and (relatively) unde-layed neuronal responses to signal envelopes have to converge on neurons that multiply and integrate their coinciding input. Different response delays were indeed distinguish-able in the neuronal recordings of midbrain neurons (see Fig. 8.9) and enhanced responses were observed when the stimulus had the right period to compensate for the delay differences (see Fig. 8.10).

But a neuronal model capable of explaining the temporal tuning of these neurons should also be able to provide explanations for other neuronal features, for example, it should explain why the BMFs of these neurons depend on the carrier of an AM signal (see Fig. 9.8; Langner, 1983; Langner and Schreiner, 1988). The challenge was met by a neuronal model which performs a (cross-)correlation between the fine structure and the envelope of a signal (Langner, 1981, 1983, 1988). This model consists of a trigger neuron that triggers an oscillator and a reducer network, while the outputs of both sub-networks converge on a coincidence neuron (Fig. 9.5a).

The model functions as follows (Fig. 9.5b). At each cycle of a modulated signal the trigger neuron may be activated by its broadband input from the auditory nerve. It triggers a rapid and short intrinsic oscillation, that is, a neuronal response with a short delay, corresponding to a multiple of the intrinsic oscillation period (for more details, see below). A reducer neuron (main neuron in the reducer net) is triggered simultaneously and therefore will respond to the same cycle, but with a slightly longer delay. Reducer and oscillator responses converge on the same coincidence neuron and will coincide provided the signal period just matches their delay difference. Consequently, as a result of constant oscillator and reducer delays the coincidence unit is tuned to a particular periodicity and therefore has the ability to code the corresponding pitch.

All available evidence supports the view that the trigger, oscillator and reducer components of this model have their counterparts in neurons of the CN: onset neurons (octopus cells) correspond to trigger neurons, chopper neurons (stellate cells) to oscillators and pauser neurons (fusiform and giant cells) to reducer units. Disc-shaped cells in the inferior colliculus function as coincidence neurons (Langner, 1988). In reality, all of these neurons are certainly more complex and have more connections and functions than the model suggests. Nevertheless, the periodicity model fulfils its task in explaining how neurons in the auditory midbrain are able to code pitch and harmony (see Chapter 11).

9.4.2   The trigger

We will now consider the functions of the single model components in more detail, starting with the trigger unit (Fig. 9.5). The model is based on the premise that this neuron receives its input directly from an array of auditory nerve fibres (as indicated by a bracket around the cochlea). It can, therefore, be activated by each modulation cycle to generate one spike at a certain phase of the signal envelope. Evidence from coincidence neurons in the midbrain of guinea fowl indicates that for AM signals the zero crossing of the modulation – that is, the phase where the amplitude changes most rapidly – is the most likely trigger point.

The function of the trigger neuron is to detect the envelope periods of broadband signals, such as harmonic sounds, and to replace the complex waveform by just one spike at a specific point in time. In this way, the periodicity of the signal envelopes is extracted while all other information is neglected. Furthermore the trigger unit has to trigger and to synchronize two sub-networks: the oscillator and the reducer. As a result, the outputs of both networks are also synchronized to the signal.

It was known that octopus cells (and D-stellate cells) in the CN respond in a way comparable to the trigger units (see Chapter 7). It was, however, not quite clear how they achieve their unique temporal and spectral properties. In the meantime, detailed computer simulations that include physiological properties, such as the conductance of ionic channels, have been studied in detail and used for different simulation purposes (see below; Bahmer and Langner, 2007, 2009).

9.4.3   The oscillator

When I developed the periodicity model I saw only one explanation for the time constant of 0.4 ms (or multiples thereof) that seems to be common to the hearing system of different species, including humans: it must be a minimum value that cannot be undercut by any auditory system (Langner, 1981, 1983; Langner and Schreiner, 1988; see Figs. 4.6, 8.11, 8.12; see also Chapter 5).

The only reasonable option for such a minimum value seemed to be that 0.4 ms was the shortest possible delay for chemical synapses in different species (the rare electrical synapses are even faster). There are quite different synaptic delays in different systems and neurons, but there is certainly a lower limit for the time it takes to release the chemical transmitter, to transfer it via the synaptic cleft and, finally, to activate the postsynaptic neuron (see Box 6.1). Analysis of electrophysiological recordings from the peripheral and the central nervous systems by the Australian Nobel Prize winner Sir John Eccles (Eccles, 1964) and others (Bishop, 1953; Stauffer *et al.*, 1976; Sabatini and Regehr, 1999) has indicated that synaptic delays may be, in fact, as short as about 0.4 ms. Moreover, for neurons in the medial nucleus of the trapezoid body that have giant synapses, the delay (at 36 °C) is also around 0.4 ms (Borst *et al.*, 1995).

We used an elaborate computer simulation to study the oscillator circuit of the model in detail (Fig. 9.5a; Bahmer and Langner, 2006a, 2006b, 2007, 2009). The amplitude modulations were processed by a simulated cochlea. The resulting responses of the simulated nerve fibres were used to drive a trigger neuron, which at each modulation cycle triggered a circuit of 'fast' chopper neurons (see Fig. 9.5a). Fast chopper neurons are activated by a few auditory nerve fibres (not shown in the figure), but also excite one another. As a consequence of the reciprocal connections of two neurons with synaptic delays of 0.4 ms, their activity cycles with a period of 0.8 ms.

Neuronal circuits of more than two neurons could generate intrinsic oscillations with correspondingly longer periods. However, since the intervals of intrinsic oscillations may be as long as 8 ms, circuits of this simple type would have to be unrealistically large (20 neurons). Therefore, in the simulation the circuit of 'fast' chopper neurons is used as a pace-maker which drives a 'slow' chopper neuron. This slow neuron will then integrate input activity from the fast neurons in a normal fashion. Since its inputs arrive at multiples of 0.4 ms, it will also be firing at a *particular multiple* of 0.4 ms, the exact value defined by the time constant of its cell membrane.

It seems that under certain perceptual conditions the fast oscillations function as a neuronal clock (see below). But, for a measurement of a temporal interval, it is not enough to have a fast-running clock. One needs an additional counter which enables one to measure the number of oscillator cycles which occurred during this interval. In a way, the *slow* choppers are doing just that; they make temporal pointers (spikes) available whenever a certain number of oscillator spikes have occurred.

Besides functioning as a neuronal clock, the proposed oscillator circuit provides other processing advantages. It is known that chopper neurons are quite narrowly tuned, which is counterproductive for neurons that are supposed to code modulated (broadband) signals. For this purpose the tuning has to be broad enough to encompass, for example, the sidebands of a modulation (compare Fig. 7.2), otherwise single components would be resolved and the modulation would not be coded by the neuron. But, although the tuning of chopper neurons is comparable to that of nerve fibres, their modulation coding is much better and even comparable to that of (broadband) onset neurons (Figs. 7.7, 7.9).

Chopper neurons are able to code the modulations over a much larger *intensity* range than are nerve fibres. As our computer simulations (Bahmer and Langner, 2006b) show, this remarkable coding property will arise only if the broadly tuned onset neurons function as trigger neurons for the intrinsic oscillations. The model and simulations further suggest that, in addition, choppers would need input from only a few nerve fibres, as is actually the case (see Fig. 7.10).

9.4.4   The reducer

The response properties of coincidence neurons in the inferior colliculus include regular intervals that are related to the signal fine structure (Figs. 8.9, 9.5b). In the periodicity model these intervals are provided by the reducer network. In response to an amplitude modulation, the phase delay of the reducer spikes is an integer multiple of the carrier period $(n \cdot \tau_c)$.

How does this work? A possible answer starts with the functional role of two inhibitory neurons in Fig. 9.5a. They are assumed to function like a neuronal 'flip-flop', a processing element that is well known in information technology. The lower neuron inhibits the actual reducer neuron, but its effect is interrupted by the upper inhibitory neuron provided it is activated by the trigger neuron.

When it is released from inhibition, the (main) reducer neuron will immediately start to integrate its input from the auditory nerve. After a short delay, during which the reducer collects spikes, its membrane potential will eventually reach threshold and the neuron will fire. The firing will then reactivate the left inhibitory neuron and the whole process can be restarted by the next trigger signal.

The membrane potential of the reducer neuron will always start at the same level, which is defined by the effect of inhibition. Therefore the integration process always requires the same number of spikes to drive the membrane potential of the reducer unit to threshold (compare Fig. 7.11). As a result, this will require the same integration time – provided the input from the nerve stays constant. To the advantage of the periodicity model, at a level in the 'normal' hearing range (> 30–40 dB SPL), many auditory nerve fibres are saturated and their number of spikes is indeed independent of the signal amplitude (Smith, 1979). The small dynamic range of many auditory nerve fibres (see

Fig. 6.7), which to many modellers is an annoying functional 'deficit' of the hearing system, is therefore indispensable to the periodicity model.

In order to reach its threshold the reducer neuron has to sum up a certain number of spikes from the auditory nerve. Since below about 5 kHz auditory nerve spikes are synchronized to the signal fine structure (e.g. the carrier of an AM signal), the delayed response of the (main) reducer neuron arises at integer multiples of the corresponding period. The working principle of the reducer, the integration of synchronized activity coded in parallel in many nerve fibres, corresponds to Wever's volley principle (see Fig. 6.9). By implementing this working principle, the reducer neuron is able to code intervals of frequencies up to the limit of phase coupling (5 kHz).

For the analysis of harmonic sounds, it is essential that reducer neurons produce well-defined delays when they are activated by spectrally resolved harmonics. Because of the logarithmic frequency spacing on the basilar membrane, this is the case at least for the lowest four or five harmonics. But psychophysical experiments indicate that under certain conditions even harmonics up to the twelfth may be resolved (Bernstein and Oxenham, 2003; see also Section 4.5). For example, if a harmonic is strong enough to produce a saturated response in the corresponding nerve fibre, or it is at least stronger than its neighbours, it may dominate the response of a reducer neuron which is tuned to this frequency. It is conceivable that under such conditions the reducer would be capable of extracting the periods of this harmonic.

Some characteristics of principal neurons in the dorsal cochlear nucleus (DCN; see Chapter 5) make them likely candidates for the main reducer units in this model. This includes their inputs from the auditory nerve, their widespread projections to the inferior colliculus (Cant and Benson, 2003), their inhibition by pure tones even at their centre frequency and their release from inhibition by broadband signals. Last but not least, just like the reducer neurons in the model, principal cells synchronize precisely to periodic signals (see Section 7.2.6; Zhao and Liang, 1995).

9.4.5   The coincidence neuron

The outputs from the oscillator and reducer networks converge on the coincidence neuron. In contrast to the other neurons in the model, they are not particularly specialized since it is a general property of all neurons in the brain to respond maximally to coinciding inputs. The coincidence neurons of the periodicity model respond best when the carrier frequency (or frequency of a harmonic) and envelope frequency of a signal are correlated and the envelope period matches the difference of reducer and oscillator delay.

When both synchronization and delay compensation are optimal, coincidence neurons will respond best. Under these conditions, the delayed spikes of the reducer coincide with one of the oscillator spikes triggered at later periods of the signal. The corresponding mathematical relationship is called the 'coincidence condition' or the 'periodicity equation'. In principle, the general periodicity equation allows for several different modes of coincidence (see Box 9.2). Electrophysiological evidence supports the condition (Fig. 9.5) where the period of the envelope compensates for the delay

BOX 9.2 The periodicity equation

The periodicity equation (coincidence condition: $n\tau_c = \tau_m + \tau_k$) was first used to account for the results of electrophysiological recordings (Langner, 1981, 1983). It describes how the BMFs (= $1/\tau_{BMF}$) of coincidence neurons depend on the carrier frequency of AM signals (= $1/\tau_c$). The neuronal network (Fig. 9.5) may be considered as a building block of a correlation analysis.

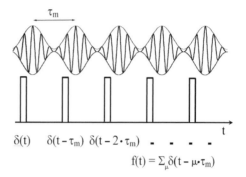

$$\delta(t) \quad \delta(t-\tau_m) \quad \delta(t-2\cdot\tau_m) \quad \text{·} \quad \text{·} \quad \text{·} \quad \text{·}$$

$$f(t) = \Sigma_\mu \delta(t - \mu\cdot\tau_m)$$

Fig. 9.2.1

The trigger neuron codes the periodicity of acoustic signals by corresponding spike trains. For our purpose the spikes may be considered as delta-functions $\delta(t)$, $\delta(t-\tau_m)$, $\delta(t-2\cdot\tau_m)$, ... Simply said, such functions cover an area that equals 1 and are non-zero only when their argument is zero (at $t = \mu \cdot \tau_m$, where μ is 0, 1, 2, ...). Together they may be expressed as a function $f(t) = \Sigma_\mu \delta(t - \mu \cdot \tau_m)$. For an auto-correlation a function $f(t)$ has to be multiplied by its delayed version $f(t - \tau_{corr})$ and integrated for each correlational delay τ_{corr} over the duration of the signal:

$$C(\tau_{corr}) = \int f(t) f(t-\tau_{corr})dt = \int \Sigma_\mu \delta(t-\mu\tau_m)\Sigma_\lambda\delta(t-\lambda\tau_m-\tau_{corr})dt.$$

The product of sums of delta-functions is only non-zero when the arguments are equal, that is, when

$$t - \mu\tau_m = t-\lambda\tau_m-\tau_{corr} \text{ or } \tau_{corr} = (\mu-\lambda)\tau_m.$$

The sum will be maximal when the delay corresponds to the signal period or is an integer multiple thereof. In the periodicity model long delays are introduced by the reducer circuit ($n\tau_c$) and smaller delays ($k\tau_k$) by the oscillator circuit. Therefore in the most general form the periodicity equation is given by: $m\tau_m + n\tau_c + k\tau_k = 0$ (τ_c = AM carrier, τ_k = oscillation period). The parameters m, n and k designate small positive or negative integer numbers. Several coincidence conditions (a–e) are possible:

(a) Usually the band-pass tuning of neurons in the midbrain obey the relationship $m\tau_m = n\tau_c - k\tau_k$ (e.g. in Fig. 9.5b: m = 1, n = –6, k = 1).

(b) Since the integer m may be larger than one, there may be more than just one response maximum in the modulation-transfer function. Such a function is called a 'comb filter' (see Section 11.2).

(c) If m is equal to zero the modulation period is neglected and integer multiples of the periods of the carrier and of the intrinsic oscillation may be compared ($n\tau_c = k\tau_k$). Pitch experiments (Fig. 5.1) as well as theoretical considerations suggest that this condition may play a role for temporal processing of pure tones or resolved frequency components of complex tones (Schneider *et al.*, 2005) and for the percept of absolute (perfect) pitch.

(d) The condition $k = 0$ and within $m\tau_m = n\tau_c$ is probably impossible, since the correlation channel coding the modulation period is the oscillator channel and therefore an oscillation delay ($k\tau_k$) is necessarily always involved.

(e) Finally, coincidences may be possible when integer multiples of the signal modulation and oscillation periods are equal ($n = 0$ and $m\tau_m = k\tau_k$ or, provided $m = k = 1$, $\tau_m = \tau_k$). This would correspond to the model of Hewitt and Meddis (Fig. 9.4).

difference of the reducer and the oscillation period, while psychophysical evidence from pitch experiments suggests that under certain conditions the variations of the periodicity equation may also play a role.

In the model, the oscillator and the main reducer neuron converge on coincidence neurons. Accordingly, the anatomical counterpart of these theoretical components – the stellate, fusiform and giant cells – project directly to the central nucleus of the inferior colliculus (Moore and Osen, 1979). In addition, their projection areas in the so-called isofrequency planes do at least partly overlap (Jähn-Siebert and Langner, 1995; Cant and Benson, 2008). Consequently they may in addition converge on the same neurons which would then function as coincidence detectors. Indeed, our experiments showed that neurons in the midbrain have appropriate response properties (e.g. Figs. 8.9, 8.10). Electrophysiological results indicate that the disc-shaped cells in the inferior colliculus (see Fig. 6.13) play the role of coincidence detectors, while the stellate cells probably have other functions, such as spectral integration of periodicity information.

9.5   Simulations of the periodicity model

9.5.1   Simulation of the components

A variety of different computer simulations of the periodicity model and its components showed that the model adequately reproduces the modulation tuning as well as other details of the temporal responses of coincidence units (Decker, 1986; Langner *et al.*, 1987a; Borst *et al.*, 2004; Voutsas and Adamy, 2005; Bahmer and Langner, 2006a, 2006b, 2007, 2009). The point plots in Fig. 9.6 show how simulated oscillator (a), reducer (b) and coincidence neurons (c) respond to amplitude modulations.

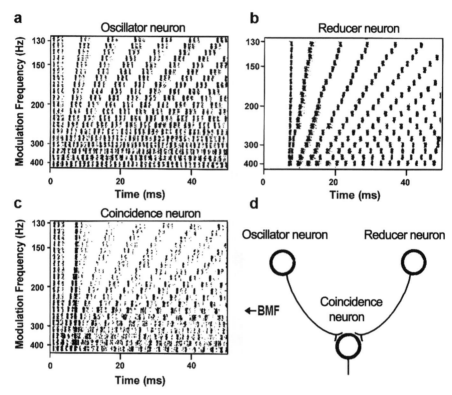

Fig. 9.6   Point plots of responses to AM signals by simulated neurons in the periodicity model (carrier 1.8 kHz 65 dB SPL). **(a)** The chopper neuron responds with a relatively short delay and transient oscillations after each wave. **(b)** The reducer neuron responds with a single spike and a relatively long delay after each modulation wave. **(c)** The neuronal response of the coincidence neuron reveals a superposition of delayed and oscillatory responses synchronized to the beginning and more or less to each of the following waves. The synchronization increases below and decreases above the BMF (arrow) of about 250 Hz (computer simulations by Decker, 1986). **(d)** Corresponding components of the periodicity model (see also Fig. 9.5).

The oscillator neuron (Fig. 9.6a) responds with a shorter delay to each modulation wave; the first spike has the delay of one oscillation period. The reducer neuron (Fig. 9.6b) responds to each wave of a modulated signal with a single spike which has a comparatively long delay. The responses are reminiscent of those of onset (trigger) neurons in the CN. As a result of the convergence of the reducer and the oscillator neuron, the coincidence neuron (Fig. 9.6c) reflects (more or less) both the oscillations and the delayed response, clearly visible at the onset during the first 8 ms. A modulation period of 4 ms is adequate to compensate for the delay difference of the two inputs. Accordingly, at a modulation frequency of 250 Hz (= BMF = 1/(4ms)) the responses of the coincidence neuron get strong (small arrow).

Moreover, transient changes in the phase delay of the reducer neuron (see Box 9.3) are responsible for the increasing synchronization below the BMF. A corresponding decrease in synchronization is visible in the range above the BMF = 250 Hz. The temporal

BOX 9.3 The synchronization effect

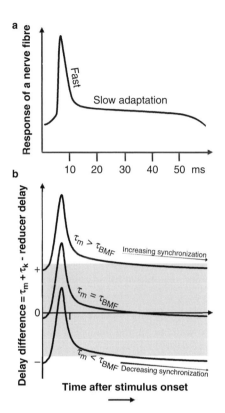

Fig. 9.3.1

As Figs. 9.6c and 9.7a show, the synchronization of coincidence neurons to AM signals may temporally decrease for modulation frequencies above and increase for modulation frequencies below the BMF. Our simulations demonstrate (Fig. 9.7a) that this effect must be the result of a temporal variation of the reducer delay, which is due to the temporal variations of its input from the nerve.

(a) A scheme of the transient response of nerve fibres (see also Fig. 6.8) shows that after an onset peak the activity of the fibres decreases, due to a fast and a slow adaptation.

(b) According to the periodicity model (Fig. 9.5) the phase delay of the reducer response mirrors its nerve input: less nerve activity increases the reducer delay while more activity decreases the delay. In the simplest case (see Fig. 9.5), the coincidence neuron is activated best (by an AM signal) if its inputs arrive at the same time. This is the case if the reducer delay is compensated by the sum of the modulation (τ_m) and oscillation (τ_k) periods.

The three curves show the corresponding delay differences (plotted on the y-axis) for three modulation periods. For the best modulation period ($\tau_m = \tau_{BMF}$; bold line in the middle) the delay difference is almost zero for a large part of the curve (after ~10 ms) and therefore the coincidence neuron would synchronize most of the time. The grey area in the figure indicates the 'coincidence window' (tolerance of the coincidence). If τ_m is larger than τ_{BMF} (upper-most curve) the delay difference after the onset decreases over time and the synchronization increases. Conversely, if τ_m is smaller than τ_{BMF} (lowest curve) the delay difference increases over time and the coincidence neuron would synchronize only shortly after the onset peak and then fade away.

gap due to the latency difference between the responses of the reducer and oscillator neurons may be seen (3–6 ms after onset). As expected, it corresponds to the period of the BMF. In summary, the similarity of the simulation responses with actual recordings (compare, for example, Fig. 8.9) shows that the periodicity model is adequate to describe the coincidence effect in the midbrain in detail.

9.5.2   Simulation of the synchronization effect

Fig. 9.7 is another example of the asymmetric transient responses to amplitude modulations (see also Box 9.3). Again, essential features, such as intrinsic oscillations and a response with a slightly larger phase delay, are discernible in the computer simulation (Fig. 9.7b) as well as in the neuronal recording from the guinea fowl midbrain (Fig. 9.7a). The latency difference between reducer and oscillator intervals is again visible as a temporal gap in the activity shortly after the onset (e.g. in the response to 135 Hz modulation frequency), while the size of this gap is equal to the period of the best modulation, again confirming the periodicity equation.

9.5.3   Simulation of the BMF shift

The periodicity model makes the prediction that, in the range of phase coupling (<5 kHz), the best modulation period should vary as a linear function of the carrier period (see Box 9.2). However, from the explanations given above it is apparent that various parameters such as the signal amplitude or the tuning properties of the neuron under investigation, will also have an effect. Therefore, in order to demonstrate the BMF shift the signal amplitude has to saturate the corresponding nerve fibres and the carrier frequencies have to stay in a narrow range around the best frequency of the coincidence neuron.

These conditions were met in the recording of modulation-transfer functions of a neuron in the midbrain of the cat (Fig. 9.8a; Langner and Schreiner, 1988). When the carrier frequencies of the signals were varied in steps of 100 Hz around the best frequency of the recorded neuron, the transfer functions flattened and their peaks shifted in a systematic way, indicating that the best modulation period is related to the carrier period in a linear way.

A computer simulation (Fig. 9.8b) with an oscillation period of 0.8 ms and a reducer delay of nine carrier periods reveals the likely underlying mechanisms, because with

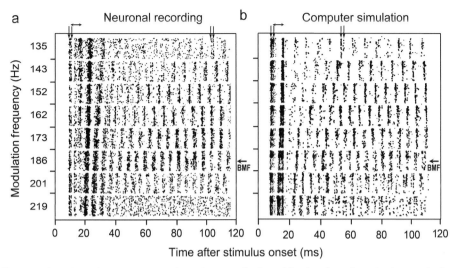

Fig. 9.7 Point plots of the responses of a real neuron in the midbrain of a guinea fowl **(a)** and of a corresponding computer simulation **(b)** to AM signals (carrier frequency = characteristic frequency = 1800 Hz; 65 dB SPL, 100 repetitions). Note the increase of synchronization for modulation frequencies below the BMF (about 180 Hz) and the decrease for modulation frequencies above the BMF (synchronization effect; compare also Fig. 8.9; see Box 9.3 for details). In this case the intrinsic oscillations had a period of 1.2 ms (= 3 · 0.4 ms; vertical arrows at the top). After a short onset oscillation and a gap of about 6 ms (horizontal arrows at the top) a slightly stronger response was elicited. At least in the simulation this response is easy to explain as follows: a reducer input needs about 7.2 ms or 14 carrier cycles to reach threshold; the onset gap corresponds to the difference between reducer and oscillator interval and, in accordance with the periodicity equation (see Box 9.2), defines the best modulation period (arrows at the side of the plots).

these parameters the shifts of the MTF maxima of the computer simulation match those of the neuronal recording. The periodicity model is thus able to explain the actual neuronal recordings: the recorded neuron acts as a coincidence detector and its response is determined by the convergence of an intrinsic oscillation with a period of 0.8 ms and another input with a delay of nine carrier periods.

9.6   Pitch effects explained by the periodicity model

9.6.1   The 'missing fundamental'

The computer simulations show that the periodicity model may explain the modulation tuning found in the midbrain. If it holds that the coincidence neurons in the midbrain mediate the perception of pitch, the model can also elucidate a variety of pitch effects and predict some new psychophysical phenomena (Langner, 1997).

Let us first reconsider the phenomenon of the 'missing fundamental' that puzzled researchers in the nineteenth and twentieth centuries (Chapters 3 and 4): even a small

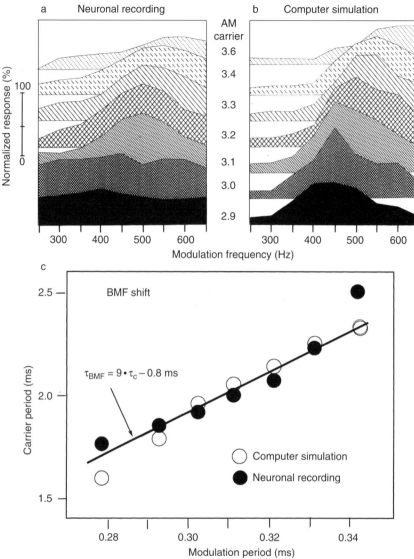

Fig. 9.8   (a) Modulation-transfer functions (MTFs) of a coincidence neuron in the inferior colliculus of the cat (from Langner and Schreiner, 1988). The BMF (maxima of MTF) of the neuron increases with carrier frequency ($f_c = 2.9–3.4$ kHz). (b) The MTFs were computed in a simulation of the periodicity model (Fig. 9.5) with appropriate time constants for the oscillation and reducer neurons. (c) Plotting the best modulation period τ_{BMF} (=1/BMF) over the carrier period τ_c (= $1/f_c$) reveals that the BMF shifts of the real and the virtual coincidence neuron may be fitted by the same linear equation ($\tau_{BMF} = 9 \cdot \tau_c - 0.8$ ms). For the computer simulation this coincidence condition has a simple explanation: the simulated reducer neuron needs nine spikes (phase-coupled to the carrier) in order to reach its threshold and the simulated oscillator introduces a small delay of 0.8 ms. The results suggest that quite similar conditions also hold for the real neurons.

part of a harmonic sound, perhaps only two or three harmonics, may elicit the same pitch as its fundamental. As we know now, it is the superposition of these frequency components and the resulting modulated temporal envelope which carries the information about the period of the missing fundamental into the cochlea. The periodicity model presented above adequately explains how this information may be extracted from the signal envelope.

9.6.2   The 'dominance region'

As the previous sections have shown, the periodicity model uses broadband and narrowband acoustic information. Oscillator neurons are triggered by broadband trigger neurons and therefore are able to code broadband envelope modulations while reducer neurons provide time references extracted from narrow frequency ranges. The first mechanism works better for high frequencies where harmonics may superpose and the second mechanism works best in the low-frequency range where harmonics tend to be resolved.

Consequently, there must be an optimal frequency region for periodicity analysis and this seems to be the area around the fourth harmonic. This prediction from the periodicity model is in line with pitch experiments where the optimal frequency range around the fourth harmonic is known as the 'dominance region' (see Section 4.2).

9.6.3   Pitch-shift effects

The periodicity equation (Box 9.2) describes how in response to AM signals the BMF of a coincidence neuron varies as a function of the carrier frequency (see Fig. 9.8). Consequently, the activation pattern over the auditory midbrain will also shift as a function of the carrier frequency and, if this pattern conveys perception, the pitch should vary too: to a first approximation, the pitch of an AM signal should be equal to the pitch of the modulation frequency and to a second approximation it must also be a function of the carrier frequency. As we know from Section 4.4, this is in fact the case.

We also know that pitch may be related to other signal components, such as to the lower sideband of AM signals or to a strong formant frequency of harmonic signals. In the light of the periodicity model, this may be related to the fact that reducer neurons can reliably and repetitively respond with the same delay to such components.

9.6.4   Absolute and relative pitch

Finally, the periodicity model may elucidate the relation between absolute (or 'perfect') and relative pitch perception. When the pianist Glenn Gould was once asked about his ability to perceive the absolute pitch of a tone without much endeavour he compared it to colour perception (Kazdin, 1989). While it remains a mystery to the majority of us, for people with absolute pitch it seems trivial to judge and, for many of them, to accurately name the pitch of a tone. Comparable to the way most of us recognize and name colours, they have neither need of an objective reference tone, for example from a tuning fork, nor do they need a special tone memory (Barnea *et al.*, 1994; Burns and Campbell, 1994). They just have to remember the name of a tone like we remember the name of a colour.

On the other hand, most people with absolute pitch seem to judge harmonic relations in music mainly indirectly, by referring to their theoretical knowledge about the relations between the musical tones. In contrast, those (i.e. most of us) with relative pitch just recognize (at least) simple harmonic tone relations without any conscious effort and, with some training, are also able to name them. I will discuss the possible neuronal basis for this intuitive ability to recognize harmonic relations and why people with absolute pitch may have problems in this respect in Chapter 11.

Obviously, the crucial point for a theory of absolute pitch perception is to explain the nature of the internal reference that is obligatory for any pitch 'measurements'. If possessors of absolute pitch rely on the periods of intrinsic oscillations, then it might be conceivable how they are able to judge the absolute value of a tone: they apply their internal neuronal clock which is 'ticking' with a period of 0.4 ms. In Fig. 5.1 we saw that a preference for pitch periods that are multiples of 0.4 ms resulted in more or less stepwise pitch shifts, providing some evidence that everybody may have some rudimentary kind of absolute pitch perception. As we have seen in Chapter 5, more evidence for some general kind of absolute pitch comes from formant frequencies of vowels, Chinese tone language and the tuning of old flutes. Infants appear to be born with the capacity to make use of absolute pitch information, although general development causes a shift towards relative pitch processing in most individuals (Levitin and Rogers, 2005). Finally, similar perceptual facilities may also be available in certain birds (see Section 5.6).

One may argue that the intrinsic oscillations with 0.4 ms as a base period may not be precise enough to serve as the required frequency standard. It is hard to see, however, where in the brain a more precise reference could be found for this purpose. In addition, ensemble processing and interpolation over many neurons may improve the situation. The fact that such neural mechanisms allow us to see thousands of different colours by means of only three different types of colour receptors (red, green and blue) certainly supports the assumption of a neuronal filter bank for periodicity information based on a small variety of different intrinsic oscillation periods.

10 Periodotopy

10.1 Spatial representation of pitch

10.1.1 Mapping from time to place

Tonotopic maps are typical examples of how perceptual parameters can be represented in the nervous system. Information about acoustic frequency is represented by an orderly topographic arrangement of neurons according to their individual frequency tuning (CF). As we have seen in the last chapters, disc-shaped cells in the inferior colliculus are usually tuned in two ways. They have a preference for a certain CF, because they receive their input from a particular location in the cochlea. In addition they act as coincidence detectors that are tuned to the periodic envelopes of harmonic signals. These neurons therefore preferentially respond to signals in a more or less narrow frequency range, especially if these signals are modulated with the 'right' (best) modulation frequency (BMF).

As a result of coincidence detection, temporal information is to a certain extent transferred into a rate (activation) code. On the other hand, synchronization deteriorates strongly for modulation frequencies above 300 Hz in the auditory midbrain and above 100 Hz in the cortex (Langner, 1992). It seems therefore reasonable to assume that the loss of temporal information must somehow be compensated for and that it could possibly be transformed into a spatial code. Accordingly, we were able to show that, as a result of the time analysis in the brainstem and the inferior colliculus, periodicity is represented topographically in a periodotopic map (Schreiner and Langner, 1988).

A black-box model of a subpart of the periodicity processing network (Fig. 10.1) shows how the periodicity analysis may result in a common map for frequency and periodicity. On the left side the frequency analysis of a small part of the cochlea is shown as a filter bank with many parallel channels (hair cells). The time information from these parallel channels is transferred with different delays via the dorsal and ventral parts of the cochlear nucleus (CN) to one of about 30 neuronal layers in the inferior colliculus.

According to the periodicity model, coincidence neurons in these layers should respond best whenever the temporal difference of the delays in their inputs is compensated by the signal period. While activation of neurons in vertical rows (dark grey circles in Fig. 10.1) of the depicted layer indicates a frequency at their CF, activation along horizontal rows (pale grey circles in Fig. 10.1) indicates that this frequency is modulated with a certain modulation frequency.

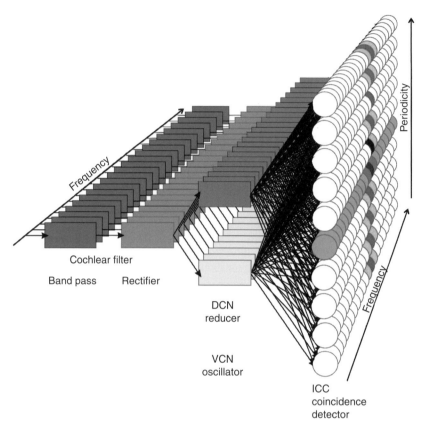

Fig. 10.1   Acoustic signals are filtered, rectified and neuronally encoded in the cochlea (from left to right; see also Chapter 6). The transformed signals are further processed in many parallel channels of which only a small fraction is depicted above. The outputs of the two subnuclei of the cochlear nucleus (DCN, VCN) converge on coincidence neurons in the inferior colliculus (ICC), thereby contributing to a correlation analysis (details in Fig. 10.5). In accordance with anatomical findings (Figs. 6.13, 6.14) the model suggests that the coincidence units are arranged in many frequency-band laminae, of which only one is shown above. One row of neurons (dark grey circles) is tuned to the same pure tone, while a certain periodicity pitch is coded along its orthogonal counterpart (pale grey circles).

The model incorporates experimental observations which indicate that frequency analysis in the cochlea and temporal processing in the brainstem ultimately result in spatial maps with an axis for frequency information and a second orthogonal axis for periodicity information (Schreiner and Langner, 1988; Langner, 1992; Heil *et al.*, 1995). The activation pattern in the neuronal lamina thus allocates a certain timbre (spectral information) and a certain pitch (temporal information) to the signal. As both perceptual parameters may be varied quite independently, one would theoretically expect orthogonality to be a feature of these maps. This simple representation allows easy and robust neural processing with anatomical connections of minimal lengths.

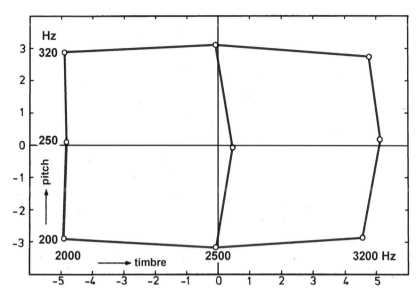

Fig. 10.2   Frequency (timbre) and pitch are perceived independently (orthogonally). The grid represents
results from a multidimensional scaling analysis: nine subjects judged the similarity of band-pass
filtered (one-third octave) harmonic sounds which differed in centre frequencies (2, 2.5, 3.2 kHz)
and fundamentals (200, 250, 320 Hz). From the observed perceptual orthogonality of spectral and
fundamental information the authors concluded that 'pitch and timbre are "independent" percepts'
(replotted from Plomp and Steeneken, 1971).

10.1.2   Orthogonality of pitch and timbre

The perceptual independence of pitch and timbre had already been quite convincingly
demonstrated by Plomp and Steeneken (1971). In a psychophysical experiment, nine
subjects were asked to judge the similarity of nine signals with three different timbres
and three different pitches. A statistical analysis of the data revealed that pitch and
timbre are perceived as independent sensory parameters that may be represented on a
two-dimensional map with orthogonal (perpendicular) axes (Fig. 10.2). Furthermore,
the perceptual distance (measure of perceived similarity) of intervals along the spectral
axis (9.62/5.96 = 1.61 times) was somewhat larger than the corresponding ones along the
orthogonal pitch axis (compare Figs. 10.11, 10.12). Plomp and Steeneken concluded
from their study that 'pitch and timbre are independent' and that timbre 'is the perceptual
correlate of the distribution of stimuli along the basilar membrane in the ear'.

10.2   Mapping the inferior colliculus

10.2.1   Electrophysiology

The black-box model in Fig. 10.1 is a summary of a large pool of data collected from
various animals, in particular guinea fowl, cat, chinchilla and gerbil (e.g. Langner, 1992,

2004). In each of these animals neuronal maps for CF, BMF, response latency and other physiological parameters were determined by recording from many neurons. The position of these neurons had to be carefully registered from stereotactic equipment while the maps were reconstructed by computer programs specialized for various forms of statistical analysis and visual representation.

According to the results from the mapping experiments, tonotopy and periodotopy are entwined in the three-dimensional network of the inferior colliculus. Moreover, orthogonality appears to hold not only for the major gradients of these neuronal maps but also for the representation within each of the about 30 frequency-band lamina of this nucleus. The key evidence for this conclusion came from experiments in the cat that Christoph Schreiner and I performed in 1983 in the laboratory of Michael Merzenich in San Francisco (Schreiner and Langner, 1988). As we have seen in Chapter 6, each lamina of the inferior colliculus is devoted to a small frequency band – probably related to perceptual filters known as 'critical bands' (Egorova and Ehret, 2008) and contains a fine structure of the tonotopic organization. In addition, the black-box model in Fig. 10.1 reflects the finding that a whole range of periodicity information is represented on each lamina, orthogonal to their tonotopic organization.

An example from the midbrain of a cat is shown in Fig. 10.3. In this particular lamina, the CFs increase from 2.1 kHz to 2.5 kHz (Fig. 10.3a), and their BMFs from 20 Hz to nearly 600 Hz (Fig. 10.3b). To a first approximation, the gradients of tonotopy and periodotopy are orthogonal. However, a slight deviation is obvious in the area of the lamina with the highest BMFs. Indeed, our recordings in the cat showed that CF and BMF are not completely independent but in a certain way related (Langner and Schreiner, 1988): although the BMF of a neuron that is tuned to a CF may vary, the highest BMF was always about CF/4. Accordingly, in the 2.1–2.5 kHz lamina shown in Fig. 10.3, a BMF as high as 600 Hz would be expected, but only for the highest CF and only in one corner. This seems indeed to be the case and explains our premature and misleading interpretation of early mapping data as probably being concentric periodicity representations (Schreiner and Langner, 1988).

In summary, although the orthogonality in the model (Fig. 10.1) is a good approximation of the actual maps, for a more complete picture further details of this organization have to be taken into account. The response to a harmonic sound in a lamina in the inferior colliculus of the cat is represented in Fig. 10.3c. The stimulus was composed of several harmonics of 300 Hz (from 1800 to 2700 Hz) and its envelope periodicity of 300 Hz explains the maximal response (white labelled area) located around the corner of the lamina where the highest BMFs above 300 Hz are represented (Fig. 10.3b).

An example of the spatial representation of BMF and response latency in a chinchilla is shown in Fig. 10.4a. All recorded neurons had a CF of about 6 kHz, while their BMFs covered more than five octaves from 20 to 650 Hz. As in all animals we investigated, low BMFs were registered more medially in the inferior colliculus than high BMFs.

The data provide a good example for the fact that not only are frequency and periodicity represented systematically in the laminae, but also, for example, average latencies of the neuronal responses to pure tones. The latency gradient points from lateral to medial and therefore orthogonally to the dorso-ventrally oriented main

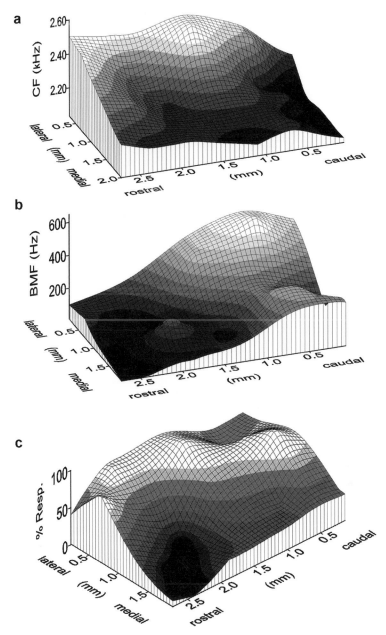

Fig. 10.3   Tonotopy is arranged orthogonal to periodotopy in the inferior colliculus of the cat. **(a)** In this particular frequency-band lamina CFs of 20 neurons increased from caudo-medial to lateral (≈2.1 kHz–2.5 kHz). **(b)** In the same neuronal lamina the BMFs increased from rostro-medial to caudo-lateral (≈20 Hz–600 Hz). The gradients of tonotopy and periodotopy are thus approximately orthogonal. **(c)** The figure shows how the neuronal lamina responds to a harmonic sound with a periodicity of 300 Hz. The maximal response (white area) indicates the area where neurons are tuned to BMFs of 300 Hz and therefore respond maximally.

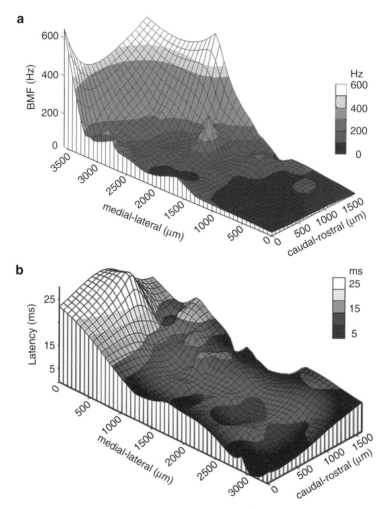

Fig. 10.4   The depicted maps of periodicity **(a)** and latency **(b)** are based on recordings in a neuronal lamina in the inferior colliculus of a chinchilla. All neurons were tuned to pure tones around 6 kHz. **(a)** The BMFs of 52 neurons increased from medial (20 Hz) to lateral (645 Hz). **(b)** Response latencies *decreased* from medial to lateral, thereby indicating that the latency of a neuron is related to its BMF (see Figs 8.13, 8.14). To facilitate the comparison the latency map is rotated by 180°.

frequency gradient (Fig. 10.4b). This seems to be generally the case in the inferior colliculus as it has also been shown in various other animal species (cat: Schreiner and Langner, 1988; mouse: Walton *et al.*, 1998: bat: Hattori and Suga, 1997; chinchilla: Langner *et al.*, 2002).

In the chinchilla (Albert, 1994) and the cat (Schreiner and Langner, 1988), it could be demonstrated that long latencies coincide locally with low BMFs and short latencies with high BMFs. This is in line with the finding that neurons which are tuned to low BMFs have long onset latencies while neurons tuned to high BMFs have short onset latencies (see Figs. 8.13, 8.14; Langner *et al.*, 1987b, 2002; Condon *et al.*, 1996). Because of this latency–periodicity relationship the latency map may be used as a basis for a reasonable computation and prediction of the corresponding periodicity map.

Other parameters have also been shown to be mapped in the inferior colliculus; these include threshold (Stiebler and Ehret, 1985), bandwidth of tuning curves and binaural input characteristics (Schreiner and Langner, 1988; Mogdans and Knudsen, 1993). However, none of these other parameters is represented in a monotonic way with a single gradient as is the case with periodicity and latency.

10.2.2   Metabolic labelling

The maps constructed from electrophysiological studies were verified by 2-deoxyglucose labelling of the neuronal response in the inferior colliculus and the cortex of gerbils (see below; for methods, see Fig. 6.14b; Langner, 2004). As an example, an image-processed radiograph of a slice from the inferior colliculus is shown in Fig. 10.5. Three broadband harmonic sounds with periodicities of 50, 400 and 800 Hz served as stimuli.

The different pitches and cut-off frequencies of the three sounds (for details, see legend of Fig. 10.5) made it possible to interpret the details of the corresponding response patterns and to relate them to the tonotopic and periodotopic organization in

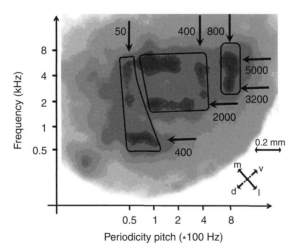

Fig. 10.5   Orthogonality of tonotopy and periodotopy in the inferior colliculus of the gerbil is demonstrated using a radiographic (2-deoxyglucose) technique. The computer-processed image shows a slice (thickness: 50 μm) from the centre of the inferior colliculus (adjacent slices look similar). The black areas show strong labelling of neurons which were tuned either to different pitches (50, 400 and 800 Hz; encircled) or to the cut-off frequencies of the three band-limited harmonic stimuli (50 pHz: 0.4–5 kHz: 400 Hz: 2–5 kHz: 800 Hz: 3.2–8 kHz; the cut-off at 8 kHz is not visible in this particular slice; stimulus duration: 1 min; presentation alternately for 45 min; 40 dB SPL). The horizontal labelling by the cut-off frequencies indicate the tonotopy, while the vertical bands correspond to the fundamental frequencies and indicate the periodotopy.

the inferior colliculus. The result is that the horizontal bands in Fig. 10.5 are due to the tonotopic and the vertical bands to the periodotopic organization. Therefore, in line with the electrophysiological studies, the periodicity information of the harmonic stimuli is mapped orthogonal to their frequency information. In addition, the 2-deoxyglucose map in Fig. 10.5 indicates that the tonotopy as well as the periodotopy in the inferior colliculus are mostly logarithmically spaced (although a bit compressed in the low-frequency range). This was indeed expected for the tonotopic axis since it is well known that the cochlear analysis creates a logarithmic frequency map. Somewhat surprisingly, the periodicity axis was also found to be (mostly) logarithmic.

10.3   'Pitch neurons'

As discussed in the first chapters of this book, periodic acoustic signals are of vital importance to animals and humans. Therefore the detection, analysis and interpretation of such sounds are essential tasks for auditory systems. Noise of all kind may blur the signal waveforms and makes it more difficult to extract them from their acoustic environment. Under such conditions envelope periodicities (pitch) help us to focus on a particular acoustic signal and to extract them from their background noise. Thus, it is useful that periodic signals often extend across a wide spectral range and that the cochlear analysis distributes their periodic fluctuations across numerous parallel frequency channels. This facilitates their detection by the subsequent neuronal periodicity analysis.

After periodicity analysis the next important step in central auditory processing must be the 'recombination' of neuronal signal components that are coding the same periodicity but in different frequency channels (like representations of vowel formants; see Box 9.1). Cochlear filtering may to a certain extent separate signals from noise, thereby enhancing signal-to-noise ratios. The main purpose of the ensuing auditory processing is probably first to 'label' and then to recombine the fragmented signal components. This latter step of processing is known as 'binding' (von der Malsburg and Schneider, 1986). From this point of view, the percept of the processing label *pitch* may be a mere byproduct of the optimization of our auditory system for signal detection tasks.

In the inferior colliculus of chinchillas, the response properties of many neurons are suitable for binding distributed periodicity information from broadband signals (Biebel and Langner, 2002). Although such neurons are often tuned to low frequencies they may also respond to higher-frequency components even two or more octaves above their own CF, although usually only with a short onset that is followed by inhibition. However, when such a high component is modulated with a frequency that equals their own CF, or is harmonically related, their response may be much stronger and more selective. Since these neurons – quite independently of the spectral composition of a signal – respond predominantly to a certain pitch (envelope period), one may call them 'pitch neurons'.

Fig. 10.6 shows the spatial and functional relationship of such a pitch neuron to the topographic organization in the inferior colliculus of a chinchilla. The result is based on a combination of electrophysiological and 2-deoxyglucose data. An electrolytic lesion,

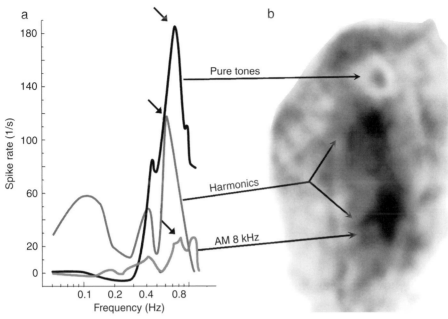

Fig. 10.6   (a) The responses of a 'pitch neuron' in the dorsal inferior colliculus of a chinchilla were largely independent of the spectral details of sounds. Stimulation with pure tones revealed a CF of 750 Hz, but the neuron also showed preferences for complex sounds with periods corresponding to 750 Hz (broadband harmonic sounds and AM signals with a carrier of 8 kHz). It may therefore be called a 'pitch neuron' for the pitch of 750 Hz. **(b)** Radiographic labelling (double arrow) of a slice through the inferior colliculus reveals the neuronal activation after stimulation with a harmonic sound (integer multiples (4–13) of 750 Hz). An electrolytic lesion indicates the location of the previously recorded pitch neuron (arrow at the top). The AM signal with a carrier frequency of 8 kHz would primarily stimulate neurons with corresponding CFs in the ventral inferior colliculus (lowest arrow). However, the modulation-transfer function (lowest curve in **(a)** measured at 30 dB SPL) indicates that the pitch neuron had some input from 8 kHz neurons: although tuned to pure tones of 750 Hz it responded even to frequencies as high as 8 kHz provided they were modulated with about 750 Hz.

which is visible in the 2-deoxyglucose image, designates the recording location of the pitch neuron (Fig. 10.6b). Furthermore, the response curves to pure tones, harmonic signals and AM signals indicate its CF of 750 Hz and its general preference for periodicities of the same frequency (Fig. 10.6a). We can see that the pitch neuron largely 'ignored' the spectral composition of the signals and responded whenever the signal had a periodicity of 750 Hz. The result of the subsequent 2-deoxyglucose experiment with a broadband harmonic sound and a periodicity of 750 Hz revealed that the recorded 'pitch neuron' was located in the corresponding low-frequency area of the inferior colliculus (compare Fig. 10.7).

These results extend the common concept of tonotopy and processing within single-frequency channels. Pitch neurons in the low-frequency part of the inferior colliculus get their main input from a narrow (low) frequency range and, in addition, they integrate over channels with higher frequencies. In any case they have a preference for their characteristic signal period (CF = BMF). In this way, they combine spectral filtering and temporal processing: they integrate and thereby bind different frequency channels that respond preferentially to the same temporal envelope modulations.

Experience tells us that somehow our auditory system has to bind neural signal constituents which are separated by auditory analysis: we *usually* hear vowels and not single formants, and we perceive complex tones as a whole and have to apply devices like Helmholtz's spheres (Fig. 3.5) to single out overtones. Also, psychophysicists tell us that across-frequency-channel processes occur in the auditory system, whereby harmonic relationships play a particular role (Yost and Sheft, 1994; Treurniet and Boucher, 2001). Further evidence comes from animal experiments: in bats, neurons in the inferior colliculus were found to respond not only to their CF but also to frequencies outside their CF area (Wenstrup and Grose, 1995; Misawa and Suga, 2001). They were termed 'combination-sensitive neurons' rather than 'pitch neurons', because in these animals they are selective for combinations of frequencies (harmonics) used in their echolocation.

10.4   Periodotopy and tonotopy: a model

So far we have seen that harmonic sounds stimulate various frequency channels and that, as a result of temporal processing in the inferior colliculus, periodicity information is laid out in neural maps. The inferior colliculus may therefore be considered as a temporal decoder which transforms periodicity information into a spatial rate code. It contains about 30 laminae, each of which represents a small frequency band (see Fig. 6.15; Schreiner and Langner, 1997). This layered network provides a framework for the representation of information about frequency (tonotopy) and periodicity (periodotopy), but also for binaural and other signal parameters.

Five of these neuronal layers are represented in a simplified model of a part of the inferior colliculus (Fig. 10.7). Orthogonal to the main frequency gradient each lamina represents a small range (less than one-third of an octave) of CF and a broad range of BMF ($\approx$ 20 Hz to CF/4). Also within each lamina the BMF gradient is more or less orthogonal to the CF gradient. Periodicity analysis, therefore, results – in addition to the tonotopic axis – in a second major neural axis in this complex network.

The orthogonality of periodicity and frequency information in the inferior colliculus provides an optimal substrate for integrating the information of broadband signals. For example, along vertical columns orthogonal to the frequency-band laminae, neurons are tuned to quite different frequencies, but to the same periodicity. Synchronous activations of neurons along this column indicate signal components (like formants; see Box 9.1) that belong to a common sound source and, therefore, are characterized by a specific fundamental frequency. As discussed above, the integration of neuronal activity by 'pitch neurons' in the low-frequency area of the inferior colliculus should help us to detect periodic signals embedded in noise.

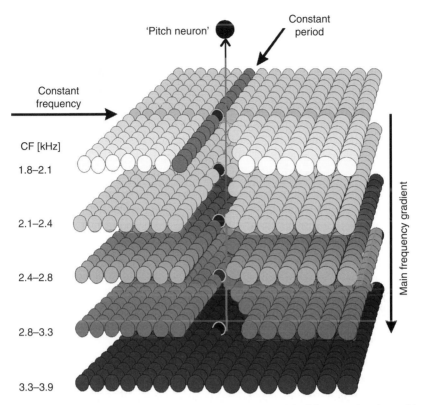

Fig. 10.7   Five of about 30 neuronal layers are represented in this model of the central nucleus of the inferior colliculus. Orthogonal to the main frequency gradient (large arrow) each lamina represents a broad range of BMF and a small range of CF. BMF and CF gradients are also orthogonal within each lamina. Parts of the laminae are 'sliced' away to show a column of neurons which are tuned to the same BMF and send their (pitch) information through the overlying laminae to 'pitch neurons' located in the low-frequency area of the inferior colliculus. The CF ranges given for each of the laminae were determined in a mapping study of the cat inferior colliculus (Schreiner and Langner, 1997).

10.5   Cortical maps

Temporal information is already degraded to a certain extent at the level of the midbrain (e.g. Fig. 8.8). One may therefore wonder to what degree temporally synchronized activity leading to the sensation of periodicity pitch reaches the cortex at all. Actually, results from neuronal recordings in mammalian auditory cortex suggest that cortical neurons synchronize only to slow time-varying signals and may be tuned to slow amplitude modulations below about 30 Hz (Schreiner *et al.*, 1983; Schulze and Langner, 1997). In contrast, in the mynah bird some neurons in the forebrain are tuned in terms of synchronization up to about 400 Hz (Hose *et al.*, 1987). Up to now, these are the maximal values found for synchronization-tuned neurons at this level and may indicate that bird brains are somewhat different, after all.

    The one-dimensional receptor array in the cochlea ultimately leads to the tonotopic axis in the cortex (Tunturi, 1944; Merzenich *et al.*, 1976; Scheich *et al.*, 1983; Thomas *et al.*, 1993). However, the cortical surface has two dimensions, which, in other sensory systems, allows for a continuous mapping of two sensory dimensions. For example, in the visual cortex, different stimulus parameters are represented in an orthogonal fashion (Hübner, 1997). Moreover, from a theoretical point of view, it has been proposed that orthogonal maps are particularly suited for two-dimensional representation of multidimensional sensory inputs (Swindale, 2004, Watkins *et al.*, 2007).

Generalized concepts for the functional organization of the auditory cortex are still lacking, although maps specialized for echo delays in the cortex of bats have been described in detail (e.g. Suga and O'Neill *et al.*, 1979). Moreover, spatial representations of various other parameters such as signal amplitude or bandwidth have been found in cat auditory cortex (Schreiner *et al.*, 2000). Nevertheless, it is now quite clear that periodicity of signal envelopes, i.e. pitch information, is represented in the auditory cortex as a major second parameter orthogonal to the tonotopic axis. Evidence has been obtained with electrophysiology, optical recording and metabolic mapping methods in various animals (Hose *et al.*, 1987; Schulze and Langner, 1999; Schulze *et al.*, 2002; Langner *et al.*, 2009) and by magneto-encephalograpy (MEG) in humans (Langner *et al.*, 1997). Finally, a more recent study in monkeys using the method of magneto-resonance imaging supported these results (Baumann *et al.*, 2011; Griffiths and Hall, 2012).

10.5.1   Periodotopy in the mynah bird

The first evidence for a periodotopic map above the midbrain came from the mynah bird (Hose *et al.*, 1987; see also Fig. 5.3). For the example given in Fig. 10.8 the coding of amplitude-modulated (AM) acoustic stimuli was studied within an isofrequency plane of the tonotopically organized Field L (CF ≈ 5 kHz) – the avian analogue of the primary auditory cortex (AI) in mammals. In terms of synchronization, two-thirds of about 250 neurons recorded in this area were found to be tuned to a BMF between 1 Hz and 380 Hz. However, while one-third of these neurons together covered about five octaves of the range of periodicity pitch sensation, most of them preferred a modulation frequency well below 20 Hz. In this range modulation frequencies are not perceived as

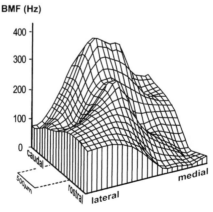

Fig. 10.8   The map shows the representation of periodicity information in Field L (avian auditory 'cortex') of a mynah bird. The tuning of the recorded neurons covered modulation frequencies from 1 to 400 Hz, thereby covering pitch as well as rhythm (Hose *et al.*, 1987).

pitch; instead they dominate the rhythmic aspects typical of animal communication sounds, speech and music. It seems that, at least in the mynah bird, one single map is devoted to modulation frequency independent of its different perceptual quality in different frequency ranges.

10.5.2   Periodotopy in the gerbil

The question arises if the second spatial axis in the mammalian cortex is also, as in birds, devoted to periodicity information. To answer this question we investigated the cortex of gerbils by means of the 2-deoxyglucose technique (Fig. 10.9). The same methods, including the broadband periodic stimuli, were already used for the investigation of the inferior colliculus (see Fig.10.5).

Serial sections of the cortex were used for spatial reconstructions of the activity labelling in the primary auditory cortical fields AI and AAF. Fig. 10.9a, b show examples from two animals that demonstrate the variability as well as the reproducibility of such reconstructions. The dark areas indicate the cortical region where neurons responded most strongly to two harmonic sounds with periodicities of 50 Hz and 400 Hz. Since the spectral composition of the stimuli cover several octaves, the labels extend correspondingly along the tonotopic gradient.

In Figure 10.9c five single stimuli labels were combined into one map by adjusting them in relation to the tip of the rostral hippocampus as an anatomical reference point.

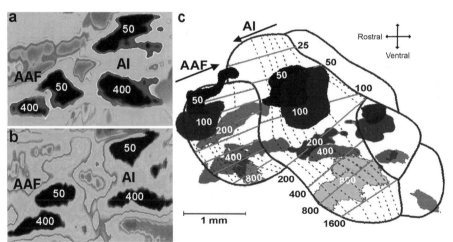

Fig. 10.9   **(a, b)** 2-deoxyglucose map (see Fig. 6.14) of responses to two harmonic sounds in AI and the anterior auditory field (AAF) in the auditory cortex of two gerbils. The stimuli had periodicities of 50 Hz and 400 Hz and their harmonics covered the spectral range from 0.4 to 5 and 2 to 8 kHz, respectively (40 dB SPL; the shading indicates the response strength). **(c)** The map is derived from experiments in five gerbils with five harmonic sounds of different pitches (50–800 Hz, only the strongest responses are shown, indicated by different shading; level: 40 dB SPL). Each stimulus had a bandwidth of several octaves, well above the missing fundamental. Due to the spectral bandwidths of the stimuli, most of the 2-deoxyglucose label extends along the tonotopic gradients (arrows). In both cortical fields periodicity is mapped along a roughly dorso-ventral gradient orthogonal to the caudo-rostrally oriented frequency gradient (see arrows; see also Fig. 6.16).

The resulting composite map shows the periodotopy in the two primary auditory cortical fields AI and AAF. Note that – in contrast to Fig. 10.9a, b – in this plot a certain shade of grey indicates a certain periodicity between 50 Hz (black) and 800 Hz (lightest grey).

The region labelled in this way represents the particular cortical area that was most strongly activated by the corresponding stimulus. The tonotopic maps of AI and AAF in this area were determined in an electrophysiological study (see Fig. 6.16; Thomas *et al.*, 1993). In Figure 10.9c only the field boundaries (continuous black lines) and isofrequency lines in AI and AAF (stippled lines) of this study are shown. The continuous grey lines plotted roughly orthogonal to the isofrequency lines approximate a logarithmic arrangement of periodicity information from about 20 to 3000 Hz. In summary, the results indicate that, like in the inferior colliculus, in the auditory cortex of the gerbil periodicity is mapped roughly orthogonally to the average tonotopic gradients (see arrows below the field names). Note that the white unlabelled areas in AI leave room for the representation of (untested) periodicities below 50 Hz and above 800 Hz.

10.5.3   Periodotopy in the cat

Nowadays, we can record the electrical and chemical changes in the brain using a variety of techniques. For example, it is possible to record small changes in the absorption of red light in the cortex; these changes reflect the oxygen consumption and thus the energy utilization of neurons. It was shown that these metabolic signals are correlated with neuronal electrical responses (see Box 10.1; Grinvald *et al.*, 1986).

By using optical recording of such intrinsic signals in five cats, we were able to provide further evidence for a periodicity map in the primary auditory cortex (Langner *et al.*, 2009). The location of the responses to pure tones is in agreement with the tonotopic gradient discovered by electrophysiological experiments (Reale and Imig, 1980). Furthermore, in line with the results of the 2-deoxyglucose experiments in gerbils (Fig. 10.9), stimulation with harmonic sounds revealed segregated bands of neuronal activation. In contrast to the pooling of data that is required for the 2-deoxyglucose technique, optical recording allows to visualize 'complete' frequency and pitch maps in the same individual. The interrelation between frequency and pitch maps was determined by averaging the response centres for all single stimulus conditions (Fig. 10.10a). In spite of the relatively large differences between individuals, the location of the average response centres corroborates the results obtained with other recording techniques. It again demonstrates that the periodotopic gradient in the cortex is approximately orthogonal to the tonotopic gradient.

In order to average the data from individual animals (thin arrows in Fig. 10.10b), the results of the regression analysis were combined by means of circular statistics. The resulting mean periodotopic gradient (bold black arrow in Fig. 10.10b; 0.65 mm/ octave) and the mean tonotopic gradient (bold white arrow; 1.08 mm/octave) were oriented nearly orthogonal to each other with a deviation of only two degrees.

Finally, it is remarkable that, in the cat, on average 1.66 (= 1.08/0.65) times more cortical territory seems to be devoted to the representation of an octave along the tonotopic than along the periodotopic gradient. Nearly the same value (1.61)

BOX 10.1   Optical recording

The recording of intrinsic optical signals makes it possible to visualize neuronal activity in the cortex. This technique relies on the fact that as neurons become activated they increase their consumption of oxygen. This is accompanied by a concomitant increase in the absorption of red light. The change in light absorption can be visualized using specialized imaging systems and measuring procedures (for details, see Dinse *et al.*, 1997; Langner *et al.*, 2009).

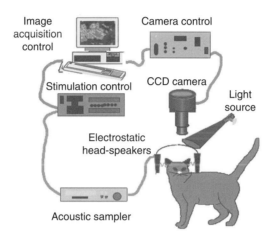

Fig. 10.1.1

Using this technique response maps for various sounds were recorded in five cats (Fig. 10.10). The auditory cortex was illuminated by red light. Multiple regression analysis was used to analyse the direction, size and significance of tonotopic and periodotopic gradients. The results of this analysis were used to average the data from all animals by means of circular statistics (Gumbel *et al.*, 1953). For that purpose vectors were added, which were given by the direction and the size of the gradients in individual animals (Fig.10.10b).

characterizes the perceptual pitch and timbre comparison by human subjects (see Fig. 10.2). This suggests that our judgement of the similarity of sensory percepts may be based on the spatial distance of their cortical representations.

10.5.4   Periodotopy in the human cortex

Magneto-encephalography is a highly accurate, non-invasive neuroimaging technique that measures the extremely weak magnetic fields produced by neuronal electrical activity, particularly that of the cortical pyramidal cells (Pantev *et al.*, 1989). The technique makes use of superconducting quantum interference electrodes

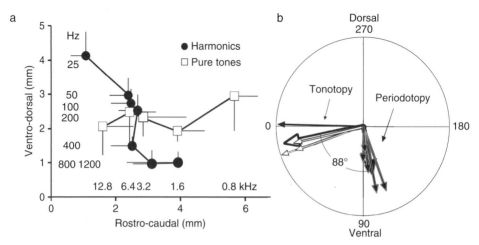

Fig. 10.10   Optical imaging signals in cat auditory cortex were recorded in response to pure tones and harmonic sounds (30–40 dB SPL). **(a)** Location of average response centres for harmonic sounds (circles) and pure tones (squares) indicating tonotopic (four animals) and periodotopic gradients (five animals). As indicated along the axes, pure tones varied in octaves from 0.8 to 12.8 kHz and the fundamentals of the band-limited harmonic sounds from 25 to 1200 Hz (lower cut-off: 0.4, 0.8, 1.6 kHz; upper cut-off always at 4.8 kHz). The results corroborate the assumption of orthogonal cortical gradients for tonotopy and periodotopy. **(b)** Results of a multiple regression analysis for individual animals. White arrows indicate the gradients of tonotopy, black arrows those of periodotopy for individual animals; bold arrows indicate the corresponding gradients averaged over all animals. The radius of the circle indicates the size of the largest gradient (1.22 mm/octave; modified from Langner *et al.*, 2009).

(SQUIDs), which provide a very direct measurement of neural electrical activity with high temporal resolution.

   Using a 122-channel neuromagnetometer in the BioMag Laboratory at Helsinki University, we studied responses in the auditory cortex of seven human subjects to harmonic and pure tone sounds (Langner *et al.*, 1997). The sound stimuli were generated outside a magnetically shielded room and were presented to the subjects seated inside via plastic tubes. While the temporal resolution of the MEG method is extremely good (in the millisecond range), the spatial resolution of evoked magnetic fields is generally considered to be of low quality. However, we found that during short time windows around the peak of the maximal response (five data points in Fig. 10.11 corresponding together to 10 ms), it was possible to localize the activation centres with a resolution of less than 3 mm.

   Up to several hundred milliseconds after stimulus onset, local activation maxima in the brain signals can be observed. In line with their latencies the maximal deflections are referred to as M60, M100, etc. Each of these local maxima seems to be generated predominantly by a certain cortical area. At these maxima, therefore, the spatial position of the evoked responses may correspond very well with the positions of their neural generators in the corresponding auditory areas.

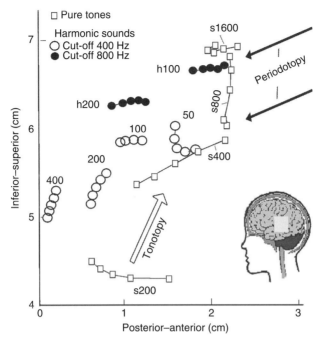

Fig. 10.11 The periodotopy in the left cortical hemisphere of a human subject (M60) is demonstrated by the positions of MEG responses (M60; latency: 60 ms; the five points at each position correspond to the latencies of 56–64 ms, in steps of 2 ms). The acoustic stimuli (<40 dB SPL) were pure tones that varied in octaves, from 50 to 1600 Hz, and harmonic sounds composed of harmonics of 50–400 Hz, in octave steps (upper cut-off frequency 5 kHz, lower 400 Hz or 800 Hz; 200 repetitions; 500 ms duration). The responses to harmonic stimuli with a cut-off frequency of 400 Hz (white circles) are located near the responses to sinusoidal tones of 400 Hz (s400), while those with a cut-off frequency of 800 Hz (h100, h200; black circles) are located near the responses for tones of 800 Hz (s800). Even in this lateral view the approximately orthogonal logarithmic representation of periodicity and frequency is obvious (adapted from Langner *et al.*, 1997).

A roughly orthogonal representation of periodicity and frequency in an auditory field related to M60 is demonstrated in Fig. 10.11 for the left hemisphere of one subject. Note that harmonic stimuli with a low cut-off frequency of 400 Hz (p50–p400) are located near the responses to pure tones of 400 Hz, while those with a cut-off frequency of 800 Hz (h100 and h200) are located near the responses to pure tones of 800 Hz. The geometric arrangement of all stimuli, as well as the nearly equal spacing of four harmonic sounds, supports the assumption that the underlying periodotopic map in the human auditory cortex is very similar to those in animals.

It is also worth noting that the line connecting the positions of responses to 'unmodulated' pure tones runs approximately orthogonal (85°) to the corresponding lines for harmonic sounds, indicating that there is also orthogonality of tonotopy and periodicity in the human auditory cortex. This result was confirmed by a statistical analysis of mapping results from five subjects (Fig. 10.12).

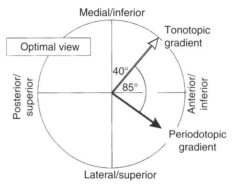

Fig. 10.12   The vectors indicate the nearly orthogonal directions (85°) of tonotopic and periodotopic gradients in MEG experiments in five human subjects, measured 100 ms after signal onset (M100). The vector lengths have a ratio of 1.3. The data are shown from an optimal viewing point (bottom), i.e. by looking from a direction in which both vectors have a maximal length. (Note that the periodotopic M100 gradient is reversed compared to that of the M60 gradient in Fig. 10.11; the same is true for the periodotopic gradients of the cortical fields AI and AAF in the gerbil, as shown in Fig. 10.9). Adapted from Langner *et al.*, 1997.

In conclusion, a total of four different experimental methods (electrophysiology, 2-deoxyglucose labelling, optical recording and MEG) applied in four different species (cats, gerbils, monkeys and humans) show that the orthogonality of periodicity and frequency, which first arises in the midbrain, is preserved at the level of the auditory cortex. The periodotopic axis could thus be considered as the second neural axis of the auditory system, as in each of these species tonotopic and periodotopic organizations have approximately constant logarithmic gradients of similar size that are orthogonal to each other.

10.6   Above the auditory cortex

Like many other experiments, the 2-deoxyglucose method showed that it is not only the different fields of the auditory cortex that are activated during sound stimulation. Various other cortical areas are co-activated, and in the case of some of them it is certainly in direct response to the acoustic stimulation. During MEG measurements in humans the maximal responses were found to jump from one cortical area to another within a few milliseconds (Langner *et al.*, 1997). Not unexpected, and in line with our knowledge about the speech centres in the human cortex, these are indications that the auditory cortex is just the entrance station of cortical sound processing which extends over many cortical fields.

Little is known of how sounds are processed at centres above the level of the primary auditory cortex. For example, a cortical centre may be present in humans where neurons are even more specialized to respond to a certain pitch (Krumbholz *et al.*, 2003; Hall and Plack, 2009). Some neuroscientists and musicologists are convinced that an important musical domain is located on the right side of the cortex, opposite to the sensory and motor speech centres on the left side (Zatorre, 2003; Zatorre *et al.*, 2007). Finally, functional imaging revealed a possible cortical centre for the temporal structure of music on the external surface of the temporal lobe (Zatorre and Samson, 1991; Griffiths *et al.*, 1998). Modern imaging and recording techniques have revealed a host of fascinating details, which unfortunately will have to be ignored here. This is currently a highly active field of neurophysiological research with new and surprising results emerging continuously (e.g. Zatorre *et al.*, 2007).

11   The neural code of harmony

'The essential basis of music is melody.'

Helmholtz, *The Sensation of Tones*, 3rd edition, 1913

11.1   The pitch helix

The pitch helix is a highly relevant concept in the psychology of music. Two nineteenth-century German mathematicians, Friedrich Wilhelm Opelt (1794–1863) and Moritz Wilhelm Drobisch (1802–1896), were the first to suggest a helical model to represent the sensation of pitch, octave equivalence and recurrence (Opelt, 1852; Drobisch, 1855).

Opelt started his career as a weaver, but later became a director of the Sächsisch-Bayrische Staatseisenbahn. Among astronomers he is still famous for his maps of the moon. Drobisch was a professor of mathematics and philosophy at the University of Leipzig and still has an enduring reputation in empirical psychology and logic.

The concept of a helical organization underlying the sensation of pitch can be related to neuronal mechanisms of temporal processing in the auditory system. Moreover, as the final chapter of this book will show, a helical organization is not restricted to mechanisms of hearing. Anatomical evidence for a variety of helical structures in non-auditory brain areas support a theory of harmonic processing of oscillatory brain signals even beyond the level of the hearing system.

But first we will have to understand the role of harmony for periodicity processing and pitch perception and the related concept of the pitch helix. It seems trivial that the pitches of two tones are perceived as very similar if their fundamental frequencies are nearly the same. Tones should sound similar, even if they do not activate the same neurons, provided they at least activate adjacent neurons in the pitch maps of the brain. However, two tones which differ in frequency by 100% (an octave) suddenly become similar again; in fact, they are often confused and may be quite difficult to distinguish if played, for example, by different instruments. Since this is true for all 12 tones of our musical scale, it makes sense to arrange them in a circle where a certain pitch quality repeats after 12 steps. As Opelt and Drobisch recognized, there is only one natural way to capture both the continuous and the circular, octave-related quality of pitch in a simple scheme: pitches have to be represented on a helix located on the surface of a virtual cylinder (Fig. 11.1).

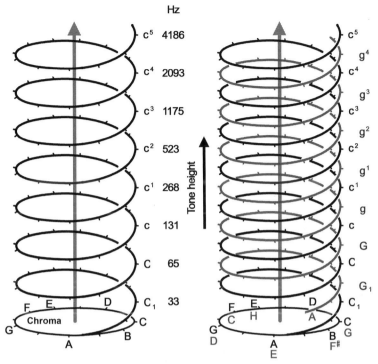

Fig. 11.1   **(a)** Each of the notes of the musical scale repeats after 12 steps of tones. Since, on the other hand, the tone height is increasing at the same time, the perceptual continuity may be captured by a simple helix. This was originally suggested by Opelt (1852) and Drobisch (1855). The chroma circle at the bottom of the depicted pitch helix represents the circularity of pitch. **(b)** A double helix takes account of the similarity of fifths in addition to that of octaves. It is similar but not identical to the one proposed by Shepard (1982), but takes account of anatomical findings shown below (see Figs. 11.7–11.12). At the bottom the figure shows some fifths as a projection from the double helix.

    The two perceptual aspects of pitch which are represented on the helix are called *tone height* and *chroma*. For example, on a piano tone height increases in steps of 85 half-tones from left to right, while the chroma (identified by the names of the notes) is periodic: after each period of 12 steps the 'same' note is reached, only one octave higher. On the pitch helix both qualities increase along the helical line, but all pitches which are related to each other in octave relationships are positioned immediately above or below each other at the same distance along the length axis of the helix. Seen from above, the helix shows only the circular chroma quality of pitch. In order to account for the similarity of fifths in addition to that of octaves, Shepard (1982) extended the Opelt–Drobisch helix to a double helix (Fig. 11.1b). It is noteworthy that a perceptual helix can indeed be demonstrated by applying multidimensional scaling to human judgements of pitch similarity (compare Fig. 10.2; Krumhansl and Shepard, 1979; Ueda and Ohgushi, 1987).

11.2   Comb filters in the midbrain

Tone height is a continuous perceptual parameter because the pitch of a tone may be varied continuously by varying its (fundamental) frequency. From the discussion in Chapter 9 we expect the similarity of two tones to be high when they activate adjacent, or even to some extent the same, neurons in pitch maps of the brain. In contrast, the chroma aspect of pitch perception is certainly more puzzling. A logical conclusion might be that the reason why two tones in an octave relationship are perceived as similar is that at least some of the neurons they activate are the same. However, this seems to contradict the experimental finding that neurons in the midbrain that are tuned to a certain pitch barely respond to the corresponding octave at a higher frequency.

How, then, can we explain our ability to recognize the octave or other harmonic relationships? The answer to this question is that – as we know already from Chapter 9 – our perception of pitch is based on a neuronal correlation analysis. Theoretically, for a certain correlational delay and a simple coincidence condition of such an analysis, not only a certain frequency, but also its integer multiples will elicit maximal responses (see Boxes 9.1 and 9.2). Therefore, a coincidence neuron of the periodicity model is tuned to a certain frequency (periodicity pitch) but should also respond preferentially to integer multiples of this frequency. Simply said, the (theoretical) coincidence neuron will, for example, 'mistake' the octave of its best modulation frequency (BMF) because two periods of the octave are equal to one period of the fundamental (see Fig. 11.13). On the other hand, by this 'error' it may indicate to the brain that the perceived tones are harmonically related.

In the equation for the coincidence condition the harmonic structure of comb filters is captured by the integer parameter m (see Box 9.2). It takes into account that a coincidence neuron may indeed also respond to a certain extent to an integer multiple ($m > 1$) of its best modulation frequency. The reason for this is that coincidences occur in the correlation network if the 'correlational delay' (or delay difference) is compensated by one or several periods of periodic sounds (compare Fig. 11.13).

Most (real) coincidence neurons in the auditory midbrain have a well-defined BMF (a preferred modulation frequency) when they are stimulated with sufficiently long tones (>100 ms). It seems, however, that at least shortly (30–100 ms) after the onset of a tone, all coincidence neurons start as comb filters, i.e. they respond not only to a certain modulation frequency but also more or less to integer multiples thereof (Ochse and Langner, 2003).

Neurons have also been found which demonstrate this behaviour even in response to longer tones (>100 ms). As an example, Fig. 11.2 shows the modulation-transfer function of a neuron in the midbrain of a guinea fowl. This particular neuron responded strongly to AM signals with a carrier of 5kHz and modulation frequencies which were integer multiples of 140 Hz.

An example for the transformation of a multi-peaked into an (almost) single-peaked modulation-transfer function (MTF) of a neuron in the midbrain of a gerbil is shown in Fig. 11.3a. The transfer function was measured in three different time windows after signal

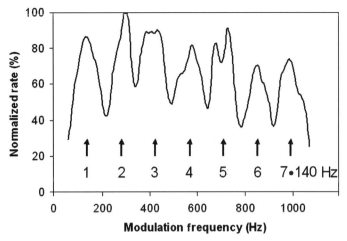

Fig. 11.2   The response of a neuron in the auditory midbrain of a bird (guinea fowl) to a modulated carrier frequency (5 kHz) reveals its comb filter property: it responds nearly equally well to various modulation frequencies that are integer multiples of about 140 Hz (65 dB SPL; modulation depth 100%; maximal response rate 35 spikes per second; modified from Albert, 1994).

onset. Up to 20 ms later the neuron responded to a modulation frequency of 220 pHz and multiples of this frequency. The higher (harmonic) modes were suppressed rapidly and by 35 ms after tone onset the transfer function could be nearly called a band pass.

11.3   Synchronized inhibition

Another example of an MTF with comb filter characteristics is shown in Fig. 11.3b. As indicated by the grey curve, this particular neuron in the midbrain of a gerbil is excited preferentially when a stimulus (such as an amplitude modulation) is modulated with a frequency of 80 Hz. However, when a substance known as bicuculline is applied iontophoretically, the neuron responds equally well to some multiples of its BMF (black curve). The explanation is that coincidence neurons in the midbrain receive inhibitory in addition to excitatory input. They are inhibited by the transmitter substances GABA (gamma-aminobutyric acid) and glycine (an amino acid). The receptors for GABA can be blocked by the substance bicuculline, a GABA receptor antagonist. The bicuculline effect implies that the higher modes of the neuronal comb filters are increasingly suppressed shortly after tone onset through neuronal inhibition (Ochse and Langner, 2002).

Fig. 11.4 shows this effect averaged over 78 coincidence neurons in the midbrain of the gerbil. On average, the responses to the BMFs of the neurons increase slightly over time and reach a maximum at about 45 ms after stimulus onset. In contrast, the responses to higher modes decrease over time, also reaching the level of responses to unmodulated signals at about 45 ms. A careful analysis of the temporal responses revealed that the

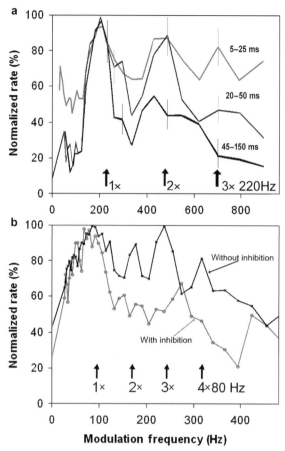

Fig. 11.3 (a) An MTF of a neuron in the midbrain of a gerbil, measured in three different time windows after signal onset (carrier frequency = 1800 Hz at the CF of the neuron; 40 dB SPL; modulation depth: 100%). The transient comb filter turns rapidly into a band-pass filter (lowest curve), which in this case is tuned to 220 Hz. **(b)** MTF of another neuron (carrier frequency = 1000p Hz = CF; 30 dB SPL; modulation depth: 100%). During a time window of 30–100 ms after signal onset, the unit is tuned to a BMF of about 80 Hz (grey curve). In contrast, when inhibitory receptors are blocked (black curve), several modulation frequencies, which are integer multiples of 80 Hz (arrows), evoke a strong response (modified from Ochse, 2005).

coincidence neurons receive inhibitory inputs which are as precisely synchronized to each period of the stimulus as their excitatory inputs (Ochse and Langner, 2003).

It is well known that the response patterns of single neurons in the midbrain are strongly influenced by inhibition (Faingold *et al.*, 1989; Vater *et al.*, 1992; Burger and Pollak, 1998; LeBeau *et al.*, 2001; Caspary *et al.*, 2002; Egorova and Ehret, 2008). Careful intracellular recordings have demonstrated that suppression of this inhibition by application of the receptor blockers bicuculline (GABA) or strychnine (glycine) both increases the responses and modifies the neuronal response patterns (Nelson and Erulkar, 1963; Covey *et al.*, 1996; Kuwada *et al.*, 1997).

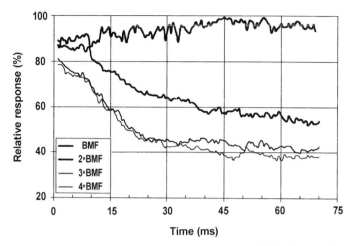

Fig. 11.4   By 100 ms after signal onset most of the neurons with comb filter characteristics have changed into band-pass filters, i.e. they are tuned just to their BMF. The figure shows this effect averaged over 78 neurons in the midbrain of gerbils. While the relative responses to the BMF even increase slightly over time and reach a maximum at about 45 ms after stimulus onset, the responses to integer multiples of the BMF decrease continuously (modified from Ochse, 2005).

It has been shown in several animals that an important inhibitory input to the inferior colliculus arises from the ventral nucleus of the lateral lemniscus (VNLL; Vater *et al.*, 1997; Covey and Casseday, 1999; Riquelme *et al.*, 2001). The input to the VNLL comes mostly from on-type neurons (octopus cells), but also from oscillator (chopper) neurons in the cochlear nucleus (CN; Adams, 1997; Vater *et al.*, 1997). The giant synapses originating from octopus cells often cover large parts of the postsynaptic cell bodies in the VNLL. This feature provides precise timing of synaptic transmission and is essential for synchronization and periodicity analysis.

11.4   The periodicity model, including inhibition

The scheme in Fig. 11.5 shows how inhibition might be included in the periodicity model. It summarizes how the synchronization induced by trigger neurons in the CN leads to broadly tuned oscillator and reducer neurons. As we know from Chapter 9, a coincidence neuron in the inferior colliculus is activated if the period of a signal compensates for the delay difference between reducer and oscillator. Under this condition, each coincidence neuron would react as a comb filter, responding to its BMF and integer multiples thereof (Fig. 11.5). The inhibition which finally transforms the comb filter into a band-pass filter is provided by neurons in the VNLL. They are activated via giant synapses either by trigger neurons or by oscillator neurons in the VCN. The temporal accuracy of this synaptic transfer explains why the observed inhibition is precisely synchronized to the periods of the signal envelopes.

The duration of the elicited inhibition in each cycle has to be shorter than the period of the BMF, but it should be at least as long as half of this period to prevent the response to

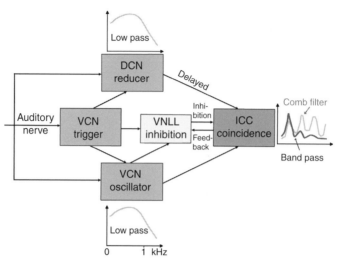

Fig. 11.5   The scheme shows a black-box version of the periodicity model (Fig. 9.5) that includes the inhibitory function of the VNLL. While the auditory nerve activates trigger, reducer and oscillator neurons in the CN, the trigger neurons synchronize the broadly tuned oscillator and reducer neuron (low pass). The coincidence neurons are characterized by comb filters which change into band-pass filters due to their inhibitory input from the VNLL (see Fig. 11.6). The inhibition is triggered by trigger neurons or, alternatively, by oscillator neurons. It is activated by a feedback from the coincidence neurons.

shorter periods (BMF/2, BMF/3, etc.; Fig. 11.6). For example, an inhibitory neuron involved in AM coding of 100 Hz (10 ms period) should be synchronized in this frequency range and provide inhibition to corresponding neurons in the inferior colliculus with a duration between 5 and 10 ms.

Obviously the transformation of a comb filter into a band-pass filter needs an appropriate adjustment of timing of inhibition. The two transmitter substances of VNLL neurons, GABA and glycine, have different time constants of inhibition. Therefore the right mixture of the faster GABA-mediated inhibition with the significantly slower glycinergic inhibition (Kraushaar and Backus, 2002) may be tailored to provide the coincidence neuron with an inhibition of suitable duration. Accordingly, the amounts of GABA and glycine, and their relative balance, were found to vary along the length axis of the VNLL (Riquelme *et al.*, 2001).

Another possibility for inhibition arises from the implementation of oscillator responses. The inhibition triggered by an oscillator neuron comes later and is prolonged by the total duration of the oscillation. Such a long inhibition time probably plays a role for the processing of long periods (low pitches). This hypothesis is in line with the finding that the oscillator neurons (stellate cells) innervate mostly the dorsal part of the VNLL (Schofield and Cant, 1997); according to the periodotopic map (Fig. 11.7) it is this part that is relevant for the processing of long periods.

Shortly after the onset of a tone, the inhibition seems to be absent, or only weak, and then subsequently increases over time. A possible explanation for this effect would be

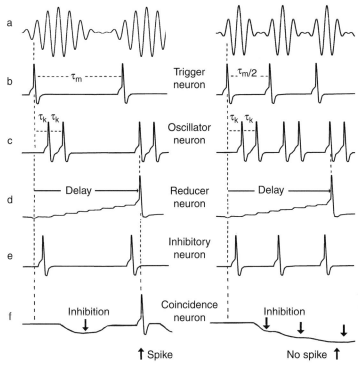

Fig. 11.6 (a) Two AM signals with the same carrier frequency but modulated with frequencies in an octave relationship ($f_m = 1/\tau_m$, $2f_m = 1/(\tau_m/2)$. (b) Trigger neurons synchronize their responses to modulated signals over a wide range of periodicity. (c) Each signal period and each spike of the trigger neuron gives rise to a short intrinsic oscillation with a constant period (τ_k); in this example, each one has only two spikes. (d) The response delay of the reducer unit is constant, since it depends only on the (constant) carrier but not on the modulation period. (e) After a short transmission delay the trigger activates inhibitory neurons in the VNLL. (f) The delay difference between oscillator and reducer responses can be compensated for, in this example by one (left side) or two (right side) signal periods. The inhibition elicited in each cycle from the VNLL is too short to affect the coincidence in the case of the longer period τ_m and therefore a spike is elicited in the coincidence neuron. When the period is shorter ($\tau_m/2$), the inhibition sums up and prevents the response (no spike).

that inhibition is only activated after the first preliminary responses in the midbrain have been elicited. After all, it would be quite counterproductive, and perhaps sometimes even undesirable, if the first responses to a signal are suppressed. Instead, it makes more sense to assume that it is only after the first signal responses are transmitted to more central processing centres that the inhibition of appropriate neurons is initiated by a feedback projection (see Fig. 11.5). An anatomical projection from the inferior colliculus to the VNLL, which might provide such a feedback, has been demonstrated in a tracer study in gerbils (Meuer *et al.*, 2003).

So far we have interpreted the inhibition of coincidence neurons as a means by which comb filters are changed into band-pass filters. Actually the mechanism will inhibit not

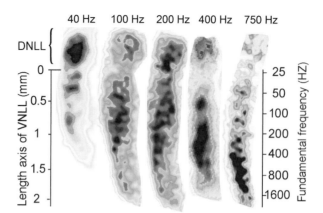

Fig. 11.7   Image-processed 2-deoxyglucose label in sections from the VNLL of five gerbils after acoustic stimulation with broadband harmonic signals (composed of frequencies from the fourth harmonic up to about 5 kHz; 40 dB SPL). With fundamental frequency (periodicity) increasing from 40 to 750 Hz the metabolic label (dark region) is shifting from dorsal to ventral. The scale of fundamental frequency (right side) reveals the statistical analysis of data shown in Fig. 11.8. The banded structure of the label reveals the helical structure of the VNLL.

only the harmonics of the BMF (of a coincidence neuron) but all kinds of higher envelope frequencies (shorter periods). In other words, the inhibition results in a low-pass filter which supports the tuning and selectivity of periodicity processing.

In more general terms one could say that inhibition obviously contributes to what is known as the 'cocktail-party effect' (the term refers to our ability to detect a voice under noisy conditions, like at a cocktail party). As the inhibitory effect on the signal extraction process is controlled by active feedback from the inferior colliculus, and possibly also from still more central areas of the hearing system, it may contribute to auditory selectivity and attention. In conclusion, it seems that the well-timed and synchronized inhibitory control allows us to focus our attention on a relevant pitch, i.e. on a signal with a certain periodicity.

11.5   The auditory double helix

The lateral lemniscus is a fibre tract which contains bundles of auditory axons from the brainstem that project to the inferior colliculus and also to the nucleus of the lateral lemniscus. In gerbils its ventral nucleus (VNLL) has an overall cylindrical shape with a length axis of about 2.15 mm and a diameter of about 0.4 mm, just the size of a caraway seed. Although they were not aware of its possible functional role, Willard and Martin (1983) were the first to propose a helical organization of the VNLL when they described the neuronal dendrites in the VNLL in the opossum to 'produce a rather tightly woven pattern that spirals in a helical manner along the column of lemniscal fibres'.

Although in comparison to other auditory structures not much is known about the response properties and the functional role of neurons in this nucleus, it seems highly likely that they might play an important role in periodicity analysis. For example, in the bat it was found that the majority of these neurons have very short recovery periods after stimulation with a tone pulse. This is in line with a special role in temporal processing, especially for echo-location, and has also been corroborated in other species (bat: Suga and Schlegel, 1973; Metzner and Radtke-Schuller, 1987; rabbit: Batra, 2006).

In all animals investigated, VNLL neurons have a high temporal resolution and can synchronize strongly to modulations of the amplitude or frequency of signals (Vater *et al.*, 1997; Wu, 1999). Often they respond to each cycle of a modulation with an onset response, which can synchronize up to 800 Hz and higher. In contrast, with a few exceptions, the periodicity tuning of neurons in the VNLL seems to be as broad as that of neurons in the CN (see Figs. 7.7, 7.9). In both the CN and VNLL, however, synchronization, the essential feature of temporal processing, is often distinct and even greater than in the auditory nerve.

In summary, periodicity information in the midbrain seems to be controlled and sharpened by inhibition, with the VNLL being the most likely control centre. Using the 2-deoxyglucose method (see Fig. 6.14b) in the gerbil VNLL, we therefore investigated whether this nucleus also has a spatial representation of periodicity information. The relatively broad tuning of its neurons results in correspondingly broad glucose labelling. Nevertheless, the responses to harmonic sounds showed that there is a periodicity map and that low pitch (periodicity) is represented dorsally and high pitch ventrally in this nucleus (Fig. 11.7). From the results of 21 experiments with harmonic sound stimulation, the positions of labelling maxima along the length axis of the VNLL were plotted against the fundamental frequency. As Fig. 11.8 shows, the distribution of data points corresponds to a logarithmic periodicity (pitch) map. It can be matched to a straight line, which indicates that, on average, 283 μm of the length of the VNLL is devoted to the processing of one octave of pitch.

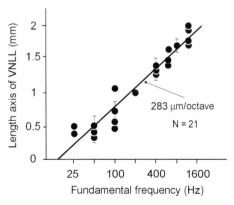

Fig. 11.8   The points indicate positions of maximal 2-deoxyglucose labelling along the length axis of the VNLL of 21 gerbils. They are plotted against the fundamental frequency of the broadband harmonic stimuli. Zero point is the minimum of labelling between DNLL and VNLL (see Fig. 11.7). The line indicates the theoretical expectation of six octaves of periodicity mapped along about 2 mm of the length axis of the VNLL.

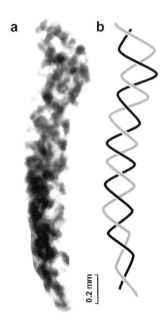

a   b

0.2 mm

Fig. 11.9   (a) The figure shows a side view of the 3D reconstruction of an image-processed 2-deoxyglucose label in the VNLL of a gerbil. In the experiment the animal was stimulated with a harmonic sound composed of eight harmonics while the fundamental was sweeping between 50 and 800 Hz (40 dB SPL). (b) The corresponding model structure suggests that the gerbil VNLL is a double helix with two times (about) six turns. The black and grey lines follow mostly the directions of highest label density in the middle part of the VNLL and correspond to the two parts of the double helix.

Finally, if one looks carefully at the label in Fig. 11.7 one may discern bending or undulatory bands that are indicative of the complex spatial structure of the VNLL. Therefore, in order to investigate the underlying spatial organization of the nucleus we reconstructed the 2-deoxyglucose label in three dimensions using a software platform for 3D data visualization (Amira, Zuse Institute Berlin, Germany; Langner *et al.*, 2003). As an example, Fig. 11.9 shows a lateral view of the VNLL, which was obtained by exposing a gerbil to a harmonic sound, composed of eight harmonics and a fundamental frequency that was modulated between 50 and 800 Hz. If one rotates the emerging 3D structure on a computer screen, the helical organization of the VNLL becomes obvious. To a certain extent this structure is noticeable also in a 2D side view (Fig. 11.9a).

The result of this 3D analysis is reminiscent of an earlier tracing study in the rat, which also revealed a helical organization of the VNLL (Merchan and Berbel, 1996). In these experiments focal injections of tracer substances into the inferior colliculus were used to study the organization of the VNLL. The 3D computer reconstruction of the resulting label demonstrated a concentrically organized topographic arrangement and is clearly in line with a helical topography with 6.5 turns (Fig. 11.10). Finally, this conclusion was

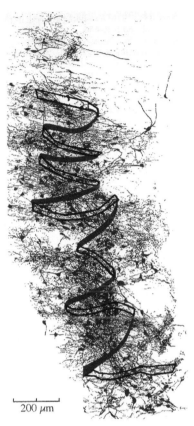

200 μm

Fig. 11.10   Side view of the VNLL from a tracer study in the rat (Merchan and Berbel, 1996). The lines indicate a helical structure which is clearly discernable when its 3D reconstruction is rotated in space (on the computer screen).

confirmed in the gerbil, where tracer injections in the inferior colliculus verified the presence of both a concentric topography and a helical organization of the cells that project from the VNLL to the inferior colliculus (Benson and Cant, 2008).

Two important aspects of the helical organization, however, only became clear after our 2-deoxyglucose studies in gerbils. These studies showed that the helix must be double and it must be devoted to the processing of pitch. The first conclusion is derived from 3D reconstructions, while the second comes from the fact that the structure of the VNLL is reminiscent of Opelt and Drobisch's pitch helix (Fig. 11.1). One may wonder if the similarity of a real anatomical structure with their theoretical construct means that it has a corresponding function in pitch processing. But the pitch map that we observed, with each of six to seven turns devoted to one octave, and the consequences of its inhibitory effect on comb filters in the inferior colliculus inevitably leads to the conclusion that this is exactly its functional role.

In summary, we deduce that the VNLL is organized as a neuronal double helix, and plays an important role in coding of pitch and harmony. This conclusion is made plausible by elaborate evaluations of the labelled structures as shown in Fig. 11.9b. Black and grey lines are superimposed over the densest label in the lateral view of the 3D reconstruction and indicate the possible constituents of the two parts of the double helix. The similarity with a double pitch helix (Fig. 11.1b) suggests that the pitches that are controlled by neighbouring neurons in the two helices differ by a fifth.

One may still wonder about the behavioural relevance to gerbils of more than six octaves of pitch. But obviously pitch or periodicity is an attribute of sounds which relates to more than just music perception and must be essential for animal (and human) communication as well. If this is true, the origin of music may be in fact acoustic communication, perhaps inter-specific as well as intra-specific.

We decided to question the human relevance of the results and investigate the corresponding participating neuronal structures and mechanisms in the human brain. Our approach was to evaluate the latter question by Nissl-stained serial sections of the human brainstem (Langner *et al.*, 2006). Fig. 11.11 shows lateral views of the VNLL from two human brains, each reconstructed in three dimensions from 30 serial sections. Although the resulting side views are certainly less convincing than the results obtained from the 2-deoxyglucose experiments in gerbils, the similarity of the overall shape and the structural details with those from the gerbil brain (Fig. 11.9a) is intriguing. The major difference seems to be that the human VNLL is larger (at 4 mm about twice as long as the VNLL in gerbils). A detailed analysis of the dense label, as indicated by the dark and grey lines in Fig. 11.11, suggests that the human VNLL is also organized as a double helix. It seems to contain slightly more than seven turns and therefore covers about seven and a half octaves, the same pitch range that is found on a piano.

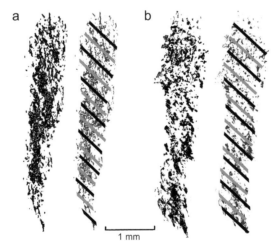

a   b

1 mm

Fig. 11.11   **(a)** Side view of a 3D reconstruction of 30 serial sections from the VNLL of a Nissl-stained human brain. Darker bands of staining in regular, nearly equal distances and with appropriate slopes suggest that the human VNLL is organized – just like the VNLL of gerbils – as a double helix (as proposed at the right). **(b)** An example from a different human brain, showing a similar result (based on material from R. Galuske, MPI for Brain Research, Frankfurt).

11.6   The neural pitch helix

The topographic models in Fig. 11.12 represent essential aspects of the auditory helix, derived from our investigations in gerbils. Fig. 11.12a is a model of the organization of pitch in the VNLL that emphasizes that each helical turn corresponds to one octave. Although the neurons are probably not sharply tuned to a certain pitch, each neuron contributes to the tuning of neurons in the inferior colliculus by providing a well-timed and synchronized inhibition that suppresses responses to higher harmonics.

For simplicity, only a few neurons are presented in Fig. 11.12a and the whole structure is shown as a single helix. With the presumed six and a half octaves the pitch range would extend from about 25 Hz to above 1600 Hz, but some cases indicate a range that may even extend over seven and a half octaves, beyond about 4000 Hz.

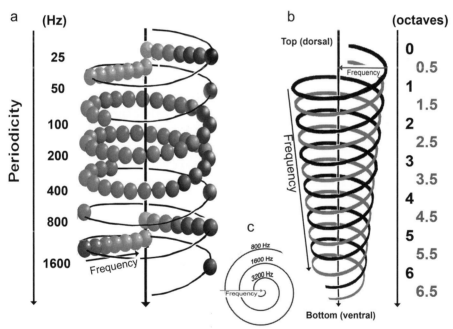

Fig. 11.12   Different experiments suggest that the VNLL has a helical organization where each turn corresponds to one octave of pitch. Both figures **(a, b)** represent highly simplified models of the VNLL and emphasize different spatial aspects. **(a)** The scheme shows the VNLL as a simple helix with only a small and (for didactic reasons) somewhat arbitrary selection of neurons. Periodicity (pitch) is mapped on 6–7 helical turns. Since the same pitch may be obtained in different spectral frequency domains, the VNLL also has a peripheral to central frequency axis (as indicated by four straight rows of neurons). **(b)** In this scheme the organization of the VNLL is outlined as a double helix. It includes the observation that the VNLL is broader at the top probably due to the fact that low pitches may occur over the whole spectral range while high pitches are restricted to the high-frequency region at the bottom. The interval between the pitches represented by the grey line versus the black line corresponds to a fifth (3:2). **(c)** A 'horizontal' section through the helix at the level of the fourth octave gives a rough idea of its spiral tonotopic organization.

In contrast to the psychophysical pitch helices (Fig. 11.1), which are just one-dimensional lines in space, the VNLL model has a real three-dimensional structure. The reason for this is that 'parallel' to the peripheral neuronal helix there are more central ones. For clarity, the more central helices have been reduced to simple chains of neurons lining up from the periphery to the centre (indicated in Fig 11.12a at four locations near 50 and 1600 Hz). All the neurons in such a chain are devoted to the processing of the same pitch. However, since the same pitch exists in different frequency domains, the different neurons of a peripheral–central chain are involved in periodicity processing in different spectral regions. This theoretical inference is in line with the finding that the VNLL, in addition to its periodotopic length axis, must also have a tonotopic axis with the characteristic frequency (CF) increasing from lateral to medial (e.g. Benson and Cant, 2008). As the highest possible pitch in each spectral range increases with frequency (see Section 10.1), there has to be another tonotopic gradient: as pitch increases along the length axis of the helix the highest possible CF at each level should also increase. These theoretical expectations have been supported by previous experimental observations (e.g. Merchan and Berbel, 1996; Malmierca *et al.*, 1998).

Another simplified scheme shows the organization of the VNLL as a *double* helix (Fig. 11.11b). In line with the interpretations above, the interval between the pitches processed by a neuron on a black line and an adjacent neuron on a grey line corresponds to a fifth (3:2). The scheme also incorporates the observation that the VNLL seems to be broader at the top than at the bottom (Figs. 11.7, 11.9, 11.11). This difference may be explained by the fact that low pitches may occur over the whole spectral range while high pitches are restricted to the high-frequency region (see above). Consequently, the upper part of the helix has to process seven to eight octaves (0.1–18 kHz or 30 kHz in gerbils) of the spectral range, while the lower part has to cover only one or two octaves (or three in gerbils).

11.7   Consonance

The omnipresence of harmonic sounds and harmonic relationships in nature is certainly in line with the basic ideas of Pythagoras: fundamental laws and simple mathematical ratios govern all realms of the physical universe (see Chapter 1). In particular, tonal harmony arises from frequencies which are in integer relationships (Krumhansl, 1990) and our sense for their harmony seems to prove that our brain is sensitive to exactly these mathematical frequency ratios.

Nevertheless, one may still wonder if it is true that, as the Pythagoreans believed, the same mathematical laws are an indispensable condition of our perception of harmonic sounds. This hypothesis is supported, for example, by the observation that a sense for consonant intervals can be observed in children prior to any experience in music and also in musically untrained adults (Koelsch *et al.*, 2000; Trainor *et al.*, 2002). Alternatively, one may share the view of some scientists that rather than being a consequence of a mathematical law, our sense of harmony is the result of biological evolution, cultural heritage, individual experience or some combination of these factors. It has even been suggested that our harmonic sense could perhaps be acquired several months before birth through listening to the harmonic sounds of our mother's voice (Terhardt, 1991). Much of the musical theory of our time is indeed based on the assumption that musical appreciation is largely a result of our cultural history (McDermott and Hauser, 2005). Schönberg, for example, was convinced that, with enough exposure, atonal music would become as popular as tonal music. This has not proved to be the case since obviously most music lovers still prefer tonal music. Judging from this, it seems unlikely that musical harmonic appreciation is primarily based on individual experience or evolutionary adaptation. It is a major conclusion of this book that our harmonic sense is more likely to be a side-effect of auditory processing that evolved for more general purposes, like communication and detection of signals in noise (see also Pinker, 1999).

In the light of neuronal periodicity analysis, we can see a possible solution to the ancient problem of musical harmony: our hearing system defines the pitch of periodic signals by performing a correlation analysis. This implies that the fundamental neuronal mechanisms underlying auditory perception indeed employ mathematical principles.

Musicologists distinguish between vertical and horizontal aspects of harmony. This terminology is obvious in musical notation: 'vertical' means that tones appear simultaneous, while 'horizontal' means that tones emerge successively. Simultaneous tones are either dissonant or consonant, with the tendency to mingle or fuse into a single percept as described by Carl Stumpf ('Verschmelzung', fusion; Stumpf, 1890). Obviously consonance has a physiological basis since even in animals musical intervals elicit regular neuronal responses at all levels of the hearing system (Fishman *et al.*, 2001; McKinney *et al.*, 2001; Tramo *et al.*, 2001). The neuronal correlation analysis makes it possible to define the regularities of these temporal patterns and thereby is also appropriate to measure the consonance of tones (Ebeling, 2008). Tonal fusion, as well as the consonance and dissonance of simultaneously presented tones, is a consequence of neuronal periodicity coding; this is corroborated by measurements of phase-locked activity from the inferior colliculus in human subjects. The results proved the preferential neuronal encoding of consonant musical relationships and a strong correlation of neural synchrony with behavioural consonance judgements (Bidelman and Krishnan, 2009).

There is still another consideration which may influence consonance judgements of musical harmony. Depending on the frequency spectrum of two tones, periodicity analysis may define not only the period of the two fundamentals (e.g. 200 and 300 Hz), but also that of their difference frequency (in this case 100 Hz) or common subharmonic. This is the percept that Rameau (1722) called the 'fundamental bass'.

11.8   Harmony

The consonance of concurrent tones is only one facet of musical harmony. It was von Helmholtz who actually regarded it as 'a mistake if consonance is considered as the essential basis for the theory of music' (Helmholtz, 1954: p. vii; see also the epigraph

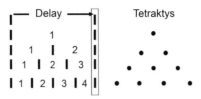

Fig. 11.13   Temporal coincidences in correlation networks (e.g. Figs. 9.3, 9.5) require that neuronal delays are compensated by one or possibly several signal periods. The corresponding scheme (left) resembles the Pythagorean tetraktys (right, see also Fig. 1.4). The musical ratios accepted by Pythagoras as consonant (1:2, 2:3 and 3:4) involved only the first four integer numbers. For the purpose of explaining all actually observed coincidence filters, as well as corresponding psychophysical aspects of tonal harmony, the coincidence scheme has to be extended beyond the number four.

at the beginning of the chapter). Temporal coding and correlation analysis may explain consonance and fusion with regard to vertical aspects of harmony (Ebeling, 2008), but they may also offer an explanation for the 'horizontal aspects of harmony', the harmonic relationships between sequential tones.

As we have seen, temporal processing mechanisms drive neurons in the midbrain to react as comb filters (Fig. 11.2). During a short time (up to about 100 ms after the onset of a tone) a coincidence neuron responds not only if the tone has a fundamental frequency equal to its BMF, but also to integer multiples thereof. This harmony effect is a mathematical property of a correlational network. In order to activate coincidence neurons, delays or, more precisely, the differences between neuronal delays have to be compensated for by *one* or *several* periods of the harmonically related periodic signal (Fig. 11.13). The resulting scheme of coincidence possibilities is equivalent to the Pythagorean symbol of harmony in nature and music: the tetraktys.

Moreover, the scheme for horizontal harmony resulting from neuronal correlation mechanisms has to be extended in another way. The reason for this is that the existence of comb filters implies that responses to a certain pitch arise not only from neurons which are tuned to the corresponding fundamental frequency (f), but also from those neurons that are tuned to subharmonics of this frequency (f/2, f/3, ...). It is intriguing and certainly important for our musical perception that, while harmonics are the constituents of major chords, a series of subharmonics amount to a minor chord. For example, the first five harmonics of C (C, c, g, c', e') belong to the C-major chord, while the first five subharmonics of C (C, C1, F1, C2, $A^b 2$) belong to the chord F-minor. This fact may solve the old problem of where minor scales come from in the first place, as musical tones (as well as most natural tones) usually contain harmonics but hardly any subharmonics.

The combined scheme of the resulting harmonic and subharmonic relationships of neural responses is shown as a matrix in Fig. 11.14. Together with the underlying model of neuronal periodicity analysis, it offers an explanation for the perceptual phenomenon of relative pitch. Note that the explanation offered in Chapter 9 (Box 9.2) for the sense of absolute (or perfect) pitch implies that pitch is determined differently in this case, namely by a comparison of reducer intervals with intrinsic oscillations. Subjects who

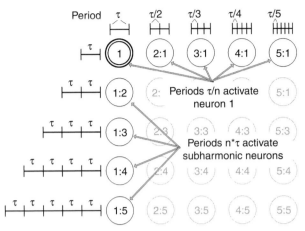

Fig. 11.14   The figure provides a scheme for both harmonic and subharmonic relationships of neural responses. The *horizontal* circles in the first row of the figure represent tones which are required to activate a comb filter neuron (1). Their periods (τ, $\tau/2$, ...) correspond to the octave (2:1) of the tone with period τ and the three notes of a major chord (3:1, 4:1 and 5:1). The first *vertical* row of circles indicate that there are ('subharmonic') neurons that would respond also (transiently) to the tone with period τ because they are tuned to an integer multiple of period τ. The frequencies represented by these neurons are the sub-octave (1:2) and the three notes of a minor chord (1:3, 1:4 and 1:5). For example if τ is the period of the note C, the two chords that are represented horizontally and vertically are C-major and F-minor. The more complete version of the matrix (grey circles) also contains other harmonic relationships. The underlying idea is that each time a certain tone is presented to our hearing system our working memory should be able to store the harmonic pattern signalled by the ensemble of activated neurons. A subsequent tone will be perceived as harmonically related to the previous one if it activates neuron 1 or one (or more) of the other neurons again.

have this extraordinary ability may determine pitch directly in a quantitative way and thereby avoid the 'stumbling blocks' of relative pitch that result from comb filtering and include harmonic and subharmonic responses. At the same time, however, the harmonic relationships uncovered in the relative pitch mode seem to remain concealed in the absolute processing mode. Accordingly, bearers of perfect pitch report that they often simply rely on their (long-term) memory for a judgement of harmonic relationships.

In contrast, most of us have a relative sense of pitch and therefore have to rely on our working memory where sensory activation patterns of activated neurons are stored for short-term use. In relative mode, the harmonic relationship of a certain tone to a previous one is established if its frequency is an integer multiple of the frequency of the previous tone. Only, in this case, the tone may reactivate (more or less strongly) one or several of the 'subharmonic coincidence neurons' that were already activated by the previous tone. Furthermore, each new tone of a sequence may serve as a new reference point for the subsequent tones or, alternatively, our working memory may retain a common reference for a whole series of tones. Obviously, we enjoy the order as well as the dynamic changes of harmonic patterns that are recognized by means of relative pitch processing and working memory.

The harmonic structure of tones as generated by musical instruments is not a product of careful manufacturing. Instead, it arises from resonances where the delays due to travel times in tubes or on strings are compensated by the periods of the harmonics (depending on boundary conditions, integer multiples of the delays or the periods may have the same effect). Similarly, the integer relationships of horizontal harmony arise –in the spirit of Pythagoras – as inevitable mathematical consequences of the neuronal correlation analysis. Our coincidence neuron would prefer certain harmonically related tones even if such relationships were not also observable in our acoustic environment. In other words, our harmonic sense for pitch relations has mathematical reasons and is not, or at least not primarily, due to the adaptation of our auditory system to the physical conditions of our environment. As a result, our brain, or at least our hearing system, reacts almost like a musical instrument and therefore obeys the same mathematical laws as the physical environment.

Perhaps in line with the philosopher Emmanuel Kant one may call our judgement of harmony *a priori* and conclude that the human preference for consonant intervals must be a universal trait of music cognition (Fritz *et al.*, 2009). However, it should not be forgotten that there are also additional *a posteriori* judgements, which probably arise from evolutionary adaptation of individual sensory experiences as well as from cultural influences that have a strong influence on our musical perception. Certainly, the extent to which we make use of our harmonic sense for tonal relations is also influenced by individual and cultural experience.

Although most of us have an acute sense of colour, some artists may prefer to paint in black and white. Similarly, in spite of our strong mathematically based sense for tonal relationships, composers of modern music may choose to circumvent tonal harmony. Furthermore, our sensory and cultural experiences determine if we prefer tonal or atonal music, enjoy Irish or Chinese pentatonic melodies or the subtle harmonies of Indian music.

12   The oscillating brain

'No sooner had the warm liquid mixed with the crumbs touched my palate than a shudder ran through me and I stopped, intent upon the extraordinary thing that was happening to me. An exquisite pleasure had invaded my senses, something isolated, detached, with no suggestion of its origin.'

Marcel Proust, *In Search of Lost Time*

12.1   'Grandmother cell' and 'cocktail-party problem'

In 1971 Otto Creutzfeldt, the director of the Department of Neurobiology of the Max-Planck Institute for Biophysical Chemistry in Göttingen, had sent Christoph von der Malsburg (Fig. 12.1c) and me – the two young physicists in his group – to the Sorbonne in Paris. We were supposed to join a neurophysiology course organized by the International Brain Research Organization. The Parisian atmosphere and the lively discussions about the functioning of the brain with a dozen young neuroscientists of various nationalities in the cafés of the Quartier Latin would certainly inspire our research in the following years. Back in Göttingen, both Christoph and I studied the temporal aspects of neuronal feature detection; I started to investigate the coding of amplitude modulations in the midbrain of guinea fowl, while Christoph worked on neuronal nets in the visual cortex, and also on a solution for the 'cocktail-party problem'. In other words, he tried to answer the question of how our brain manages to isolate a particular voice under the noisy conditions of a cocktail party (see Chapter 6). But in his paper entitled 'A neural cocktail-party processor' the acoustic example of feature analysis served only as a pertinent example for the more general 'binding problem' (von der Malsburg and Schneider, 1986).

It is obvious that not only the auditory but all sensory systems have to coordinate features distributed over space and time – features like size, position, direction and colour in vision or loudness, position, pitch and timbre in hearing. Usually our brain has to organize coherent neural representations and processing streams which are related to multisensory features. Nevertheless, it usually manages to provide us with a unity of experience. For this purpose our brain has to decide which neuronal activations actually belong together and which belong to different objects. The idea was that all features of a pattern or a Gestalt, which were collected and represented by specialized feature detector cells in the brain, are combined in the inputs of highly specialized neurons. Their activation would then perhaps signal a certain person, a particular object or a specific event.

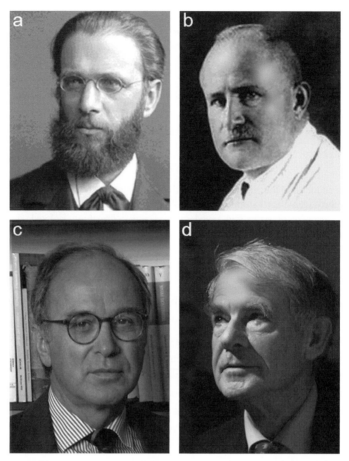

Fig. 12.1   **(a)** Carl Stumpf (1848–1936) was regarded as one of the greatest scientists of his time. He was influential in the fields of philosophy and psychology, as well as musicology, around the turn of the century. At the organ in the cathedral in Halle (Saxony) he investigated the psychological phenomenon of 'Verschmelzung' (fusion). **(b)** The physician and scientist Hans Berger (1873–1941) was the director of the Psychiatric Clinic in Jena. He discovered brain waves and developed the first method for the recording and graphical representation of the electro-encephalogram (EEG). **(c)** The physicist and neuroscientist Christoph von der Malsburg started his career in 1972 in Otto Creutzfeldt's department at the Max-Planck Institute in Göttingen. In 1983 he suggested synchrony coding as a solution for the neural binding problem and thus marked the beginning of a new research era. **(d)** The neuroscientist Wolf Singer started his career in 1968 in Otto Creutzfeldt's department at the University of München, addressing the problem of EEG synchrony. As director of the Max-Planck Institute for Brain Research in Frankfurt, he demonstrated that the synchronization of neuronal oscillations is adequate to bind visual and other signals distributed over the cortex.

This concept was originally addressed by the term 'grandmother cell', a hypothetical neuron that would be highly selective for a certain complex signal such as the face or the voice of one's grandmother (Lettvin *et al.*, 1959; Bullock, 1961; Gross, 2002). It immediately raised a lot of new questions: Are there enough selective cells to represent all the people and objects we have ever learned to recognize? Will there be enough new cells available for every new object? Don't we also recognize grandma on the telephone when no visual features are available? These are just a few questions evoked by this concept (for more details, see von der Malsburg, 1999). As a matter of fact, highly specialized neurons were indeed found in a cortical area devoted to face recognition (Rolls *et al.*, 2006), but even these cells were not as selective as expected theoretically from a real 'grandmother cell'. On the other hand, if such cells are not the solution for binding associated features, another processing strategy would be necessary.

The strategy Christoph came up with was – similar to the periodicity theory (Chapter 9) – based on neuronal oscillation and synchronization. Neurons which fire in a highly synchronized way, with the same frequency and a constant phase relationship, are very likely to belong to the same neuronal ensemble or net. They respond in this way to their inputs because they are directly or indirectly connected in a specific way by synapses which may underlie plastic changes. Previous repetitive stimulations of these synapses gave rise to plastic modifications and thereby established the neuronal net as a memory trace (representation) of the stimulus. If the brain were able to evaluate which neurons actually participate in a synchronized oscillation, the binding problem would be solved and the 'grandmother' recognized.

12.2   Binding and oscillations

12.2.1   A historical note

In the late nineteenth century, about 100 years before von der Malsburg theorized about cocktail-party processing, the hypothesis of neural oscillations was put forward independently by T. H. Huxley (1880) and by Henry Maudsley (1884). They expanded the ideas of the Yorkshire philosopher and psychologist David Hartley (1705–1757), who had realized that our perception must be based on some kind of nerve vibrations since it may 'last for a while' after a corresponding stimulation. Hartley agreed with corresponding speculations in Isaac Newton's *Principia* (1723), which in turn were inspired by Kepler's and Pythagoras' ideas about world harmony (wikipedia.org/wiki/David_Hartley; also see Chapter 1).

At the same time as Huxley and Maudsley wrote their books, the famous philosopher and psychologist Carl Stumpf (1848–1936; Fig. 12.1a) used the organ of the Dom in Halle in Saxony to investigate a psychological phenomenon which he called fusion ('Verschmelzung'; Stumpf, 1890; Ebeling, 2008). Basically, this term stands for the way our brains tend to fuse or bind different but related fundamental percepts. Fusion is a well-known phenomenon and quite obvious in the case of several simple tones which together build a harmonic sound or a musical chord. This is especially true for tones an octave apart that tend to fuse and subsequently are difficult or even impossible to separate. To a lesser extent this is also true for other harmonic intervals, such as fifths or thirds. The phenomenon of fusion indicates that the binding of oscillating neurons in the brain may not necessarily be restricted to a particular frequency but may also encompass harmonically related frequencies (Glassman, 1999). Moreover, as Stumpf realized, this effect is not limited to hearing nor to one modality alone; it helps us to recognize complex objects (Gestalten) of all kinds, such as melodies or grandmothers, and relate these to our memories and emotions.

Until the early twentieth century nobody knew of the actual existence of brain oscillations, not to mention that it would be actually possible to measure them. It was in 1924 in Jena, some 50 miles from Halle, where the neurologist Hans Berger (1873–1941; Fig. 12.1b) first recorded electrical 'rhythms' from the human scalp. Although he used a string galvanometer, his simple electro-encephalographic (EEG) technique allowed him to recognize if his subject was awake or sleeping. Suffering from depression, Berger killed himself in the summer of 1941 and his pioneering discovery, although nominated several times, had to remain uncrowned with the Nobel Prize.

Nowadays the EEG is a standard clinical technique and brain waves have been located to motor and sensory cortices, as well as association and control structures (Başar *et al.*, 2001; Brosch *et al.*, 2002). It is now well known that many cognitive and behavioural aspects of brain processing are intimately linked to brain oscillations (Schroeder and Lakatos, 2009). While slow oscillations are known to play a role in the consolidation of memories during sleep (Born and Wagner, 2004), fast gamma-oscillations are involved in attention, short-term memory and conscious awareness (Born *et al.*, 2006).

Because of their different physiological and behavioural significance, the frequency range of brain waves is divided into delta, theta, alpha, beta and gamma bands, extending over the range from about 2 to 250 Hz. Since there is no common agreement in neuroscience about the exact frequency boundaries of these bands, Fig. 12.2 suggests a subdivision into octaves (see also Glassman, 1999), which, in correspondence to the pitch helix (see Fig. 11.1), are mapped here on a helix with seven turns.

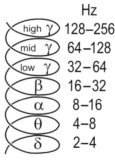

Hz

high γ	128–256
mid γ	64–128
low γ	32–64
β	16–32
α	8–16
θ	4–8
δ	2–4

Fig. 12.2   Brain oscillations extend over approximately seven octaves from about 2 to 250 Hz, mapped here on a helix. Rising from low to high frequencies, each octave may be roughly related to a major physiological function: delta (δ) to deep sleep, theta (θ) to drowsiness or meditation, alpha (α) to open eyes and wakefulness, beta (β) to alertness and movements and gamma (γ) to active thinking and concentration.

In humans, oscillations of the brain are usually recorded with electrodes on the surface of the head. The measured potentials result from the interference of the electrical activity of many thousands, or perhaps even millions, of neurons. Nevertheless, they give rise to only noisy signals in the microvolt range that allow no more than a rough insight into brain mechanisms. Better results can be obtained with electrodes directly contacting the brain surface, but for medical and ethical reasons this method is necessarily confined to certain patients. In contrast, the use of surface as well as depth electrodes in experimental animals permits better recordings that allow one to answer more sophisticated questions.

With experiments of this kind another of Otto Creutzfeldt's scholars, Wolf Singer (Fig. 12.1d), started his career in 1968 at the University of Munich. Soon after becoming the director of the Max-Planck Institute for Brain Research in Frankfurt, Singer and his group started to investigate synchronized neuronal responses. The results of this research, which initially concentrated on the visual cortex, surprised and amazed the neurophysiological community. By recording from cortical neurons, Singer and other neuroscientists (Eckhorn *et al.*, 1988; Gray *et al.*, 1990; Singer, 1999, 2001, 2007) were able to demonstrate that the synchronized activity of neuronal oscillations, especially in the so-called gamma band (>30 Hz), could be adequate to bind different aspects of visual and other sensory signals (Gray, 1999). For example, neurons in two separated areas of the cortex, each tuned to a moving bar in its own receptive field, were demonstrated to synchronize when stimulated by a large common bar. Their synchronization was shown to be a network property and the synchronized neurons could be separated by many millimetres or even located on opposite sides of the brain (Eckhorn *et al.*, 1988; Engel and Singer, 2001). Furthermore, experiments in awake, behaving animals (Fries *et al.*, 2001; Fries, 2009) indicated that neuronal synchronization in the gamma band may even be a necessary prerequisite for conscious perception. This was the conclusion from the observation that neurons tuned to a particular feature of a visual stimulus were synchronized whenever the animal responded with a certain behavioural reaction to this feature.

12.2.2   Binding and neuronal correlation analysis

Mechanisms of processing comparable to those in the hearing system seem to be required for the binding of visual images and the fusion of incidents in all sensory and non-sensory modalities. One might therefore expect to find trigger neurons, which are able to pick up transient and especially periodic events, as well as oscillatory, integrative or delay mechanisms that provide exact timing signals for correlational purposes.

The demonstration of these processing components is not possible without thorough electrophysiological investigations, and an understanding of their functional interactions may not be accessible without appropriate modelling. On the other hand, bearing in mind the anatomical rule 'form follows function', one might expect to find structures in appropriate anatomical preparations in a form which indicates their function. In the auditory system this is the case for the ventral nucleus of the lateral lemniscus (VNLL). Its helical appearance indicates its functional role as a control device for several octaves of acoustic frequencies and its involvement in the binding of harmonically related signal components. In conclusion, if the processing of oscillations is comparable in other areas of the brain beyond the hearing system, one might perhaps expect to see similar helical structures in non-auditory areas.

The inhibitory control in the auditory system seems to be mostly an 'automatic' bottom-up process driven mostly by the amplitude of periodic input signals, but there are also top-down mechanisms which allow us to direct our attention and to adjust this automatic processing. Probably, this is the main purpose of the strong efferent projections of neurons from the deep layers of the auditory cortex to the geniculate body, the midbrain and even lower auditory nuclei (Suga et al., 2000). It seems certain that the harmonic sound processor in the VNLL, with its helical anatomical design and its inhibitory control of (and feedback from) the inferior colliculus, is another key player in this game. The idea of inhibitory control of oscillations in periodicity processing is in line with computer simulations of the visual cortex which showed that an increase in synchronized inhibition could enhance neuronal oscillations and thus also visual attention (Tiesinga et al., 2004; Singer, 2013).

Helical structures may be found in many different biological systems, with the DNA double helix and the structure of many proteins being the best-known examples. From this perspective it may be surprising that the only neuronal helix described so far in the brain is the VNLL, in spite of the fact that single stained sections of a variety of brain structures may look quite similar – with the most striking examples coming from the limbic system, the basal ganglia and the reticular formation (Figs. 12.4–12.8). Fig. 12.3 depicts their approximate location in the human brain. However, as is also true for the VNLL, only thorough anatomical investigations including 3D reconstructions can show to what extent these structures really are helically organized and careful physiological studies are required to elucidate the potential role of such seemingly helical structures.

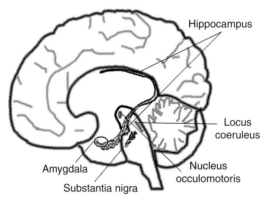

Fig 12.3   This sagittal section through the human brain shows the location of neuronal structures which bear some resemblance to the helical VNLL. The helical-like structures either belong to the basal ganglia (substantia nigra), reticular formation (locus coeruleus) or the limbic system (hippocampus and amygdala).

12.3   Helical brain structures

12.3.1   The 'blue' helix

The locus coeruleus (LC) or 'blue spot' is a spindle-like structure in the reticular formation of the brainstem. Although in humans the LC is only about 12 mm long and 1–2 mm wide, it contains about 12 000 neurons which are characterized by a high content of the inhibitory neurotransmitter noradrenaline. With their widespread branched axons, the neurons of the LC project to every major region of the brain: the forebrain, thalamic nuclei, hippocampus, hypothalamus, cerebellum and spinal cord.

The LC is involved in a variety of physiological processes and plays an important role in all kinds of behaviour. By means of its inhibitory synapses it amplifies relevant signals and enhances signal-to-noise ratios in the target centres. The role of the LC in the regulation of the stages of sleep, where neurons may fire only one or two spikes per second, is well known. In contrast, during waking and attention the frequency of neuronal oscillatory activity of the LC may increase by several octaves. Accordingly, electrical stimulation of the LC in the cat facilitates oscillatory activity in the gamma frequency range and enhances the synchronization of neuronal oscillations in the visual cortex (Munk *et al.*, 1996). Indeed, the control of mood, arousal, attention and sexual behaviour relies on the proper functioning of the LC.

Fig 12.4a shows one section through the LC of a human brainstem, which was stained with the Nissl staining technique. Each little black dot in this image, as well as in the 3D

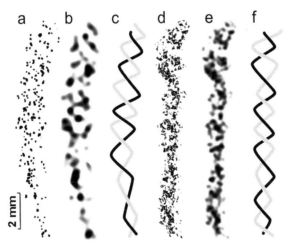

Fig 12.4   (a) A Nissl-stained coronal section through the human locus coeruleus (material courtesy of R. Galuske, MPI for Brain Research, Frankfurt). Each black dot in the figure corresponds to a single neuron. Note the bands of aligned neurons, which are usually called 'columns'. (b) The same section, but the image has been heavily blurred. (c) An 'artistic' interpretation of the helical appearance of the 3D reconstruction, which is even more obvious when the image is rotated on the computer monitor. (d) A side view of a 3D reconstruction of the same structure from a series of parallel sections. (e) The same section, but the image has been blurred. (f) The figure shows that the locus coeruleus may be interpreted as a double helix with more than five turns.

reconstruction, represents a single labelled cell (fusions of several dots are due to image processing). Although slightly larger, the LC looks strikingly similar to the helical VNLL (see Figs. 11.9, 11.11). This holds not only for its overall spindle-like shape, but also for the banded structure of aligned neurons which anatomists call 'columns'. If one makes a 3D reconstruction by combining several brain slices (Fig 12.4b), the similarity becomes even more obvious (especially when rotated on a computer screen). Consequently, the LC is interpreted here as a double helix with more than five turns (Fig. 12.4c,f).

The similarity of the LC with the VNLL suggests that its function may also be comparable; its more than five turns may be involved in the control of EEG waves from about delta to mid-gamma or from theta to high-gamma (compare Fig. 12.2). This implies that its proper activation could enhance a particular oscillation frequency and suppress competing ones. Thus, the LC may indeed act as a temporal attentional filter that selectively facilitates task-relevant behaviours (Aston-Jones and Cohen, 2005). As a consequence we would be able to pay attention to any perceptual, cognitive or emotional item that is represented by a particular oscillation frequency or a combination of (harmonically) related frequencies. As we will discuss below, such attentional tasks probably involve synchronization of different brain waves in various brain areas (Singer, 2013; see Fig. 12.9). The tiny LC with its widespread inhibitory control of every major region of the brain seems to have just the right anatomical and functional properties for this purpose.

12.3.2   The helix for eye movement

We constantly and rapidly rotate our eyes using three pairs of small muscles. The reason is that the fovea centralis, the only location of really sharp vision on our retina, is tiny and covers only a few degrees of our visual field. By means of the eye movements (saccades) we scan the visual field and move this spot in different directions at different speeds. Nevertheless, we usually have the impression of a stable visual environment. A possible explanation is that oscillations are triggered each time we look at a particular point. These oscillations continue for a short time and establish a stable representation of the visual image in our working memory.

Due to the deficits in their dopamine receptor system, schizophrenic patients have problems controlling oscillations (Grace, 1991; Uhlhaas *et al.*, 2008). They may be interrupted too quickly and, in the visual system, the image of the environment is fragmented into small pieces, as patients actually report (Whittington and Traub, 2003). On the other hand, not only in the visual system, the deficit may result in uncontrolled, persistent oscillations, which probably explains symptoms such as hallucinations or hearing voices.

How our image-scanning eyes are coordinated and synchronized with the image-processing parts of our brain is only partly understood. Several brain areas are involved in controlling the movement of the eyes and coordinating them with trigger signals arriving from different sensory modalities. For example, the superior colliculus (neighbouring the inferior colliculus) contains topographically organized neurons which

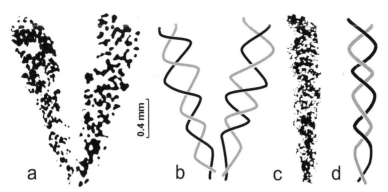

Fig 12.5   (a, b) The left and right oculomotor nuclei of a human brain resemble the helical VNLL. (c) Graphic interpretation of their helical appearance. Left oculomotor nuclei of another human brain and its graphic interpretation (d) (material from R. Galuske, MPI for Brain Research, Frankfurt).

control the direction and velocity of eye saccades. Its main input comes from the eyes, but there are also other sensory triggers, such as an auditory one from the inferior colliculus. A top-down control from a cortical executive centre may select appropriate saccades and trigger voluntary ones. Their direction depends on oscillations in the frequency range between 25 and 90 Hz that are synchronized with corresponding cortical oscillations (Pesaran, 2002).

Fig. 12.5a shows the Nissl-stained sections of the left and right oculomotor nuclei of a human brain. Moreover, the graphic interpretation in Fig. 12.5b suggests a conical structure, which is reminiscent of a double helix with about three turns. Fig. 12.5c shows the left oculomotor nuclei of another human brain and Fig. 12.5d the corresponding graphic interpretation. In both cases the oculomotor nucleus is structurally similar to the VNLL. Assuming a similar function, this suggests a control of neuronal oscillation frequency over about three octaves, which could include the two octaves from 25 to 100 Hz (see above).

12.3.3   The helix of emotion

Odours have an especially intense effect on emotions and memory – we have all experienced this at some point. One of the opening scenes in Marcel Proust's novel *In Search of Lost Time* is an example of how the amygdala receives input from the olfactory system; the sensations experienced by Proust by simply sipping tea and tasting a piece of cake, a Madeleine, were sufficient to evoke intense memories of his childhood and induce a wonderful rush of happiness. In music psychology, such surprising emotional experiences are described as 'musical chills'. One may experience this sensation when a piece of music evokes a pleasant, although perhaps subliminal, memory.

The limbic system, which runs through the entire brain, is important for the processing of such intense emotions. Although often treated as one brain structure,

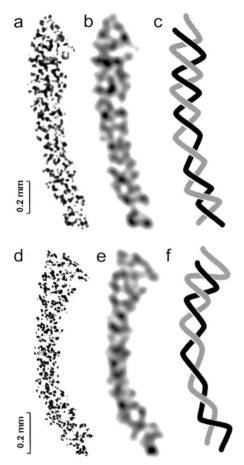

Fig 12.6   Single sections through a Nissl-stained substructure of the amygdala of a rat **(a)** and a mouse **(d)**. Again, each dot in these images corresponds to a single neuron (fusion into larger dots and stripes is due to image processing). **(b, e)** Blurring the images enhances their overall helical appearance. **(c, f)** The graphic interpretations suggest helical structures, i.e. double helices with five to six turns (brain sections from http://brainmaps.org).

it includes the hippocampus and the amygdala (Greek for 'almond'), which itself consists of various subnuclei. The amygdala complex is interconnected with all major parts of the brain and it receives all of the important sensory information. Accordingly, its main function seems to be to generate and control emotions and to ensure emotional learning (LeDoux, 1992; Aggleton, 1993). It is also involved with the generation of anxiety, which is a necessary part of normal functioning for producing appropriate defence and flight behaviour. However, when it malfunctions, symptoms such as memory disorders, emotional deficits and depression may become apparent (Reinhold *et al.*, 2006).

Fig. 12.6 shows Nissl-stained sections through the ventro-lateral nucleus of the amygdala complex of a rat (a–c) and of a mouse (d–f). The underlying structure becomes more obvious in the corresponding blurred images (b,e). The graphic interpretations (c,f) and the obvious resemblance to the VNLL suggest that the amygdala contains a substructure which is helically organized. The figures suggest that this structure is organized as a double helix which – at least in rat and mouse – has about six turns.

A helix in the amygdala would imply that frequencies, as well as harmonic relations of brain waves, are related to or have an impact on emotions. Indeed, the frequencies of brain oscillations are known to be related to activation or arousal, from calmness to excitement. For example, it is known that alpha waves are typical for an alert but relaxed mental state of mind, while beta waves are related to a more active state. On the other hand, very low frequencies are typical for sadness and depression while high frequencies are related to joy and also anger.

12.3.4   The helical web of memory

Another important and fascinating structure in the limbic system is the hippocampus (HC). Located in the centre of the brain, this structure plays a crucial role in episodic memory storage and also in the retrieval of memory information. New incoming information activates the HC, which somehow supports the activity-dependent plastic changes of synapses that serve as storage devices in nets or assemblies of cortical neurons (Hebb, 1961). These neuronal nets for memory seem to be distributed over the whole cortex, including the parts of the sensory cortex that provided the original input.

If our hippocampus were damaged or destroyed, we would still have a short-term memory but we would not be able to keep anything in mind for more than a few minutes. Important or unimportant, everything would be forgotten completely and forever. On the other hand, older memories would still be available, so the HC cannot be the final location of their storage.

An essential part of the hippocampus is called the Ammon's horn or, in Latin, *cornu ammonis* (CA); it consists of four sub-regions CA1 to CA4. Of these, CA3 seems to play a central role as its neurons receive all ongoing memory information and pass it to the cortex and many other important brain structures via the neurons in CA1. For example, in rats which have learned to navigate in a maze, gamma oscillations from CA3 were found to strongly synchronize to oscillations in CA1. This control function of CA3 was suggested as a physiological mechanism for the retrieval of HC-dependent memories (Montgomery and Buzsáki, 2007).

The appearance of CA3 in the Nissl-stained hippocampus of a gerbil is depicted in Fig. 12.7a, together with a 3D reconstruction (Fig. 12.7b) of a series of sections. Five of these sections are shown in Fig. 12.7c-1, each one accompanied by a corresponding blurred version (Fig. 12.7c-2) that emphasizes its overall appearance. The results from this analysis are shown in Fig. 12.7c-3 as graphic interpretations. These interpretations imply that CA3 has a double-helical organization. It is obvious, however, from Fig. 12.7b that CA3 cannot be just a 'simple' double helix. Instead – if the interpretation holds – the hippocampus seems to contain a network with dozens of parallel double-helices.

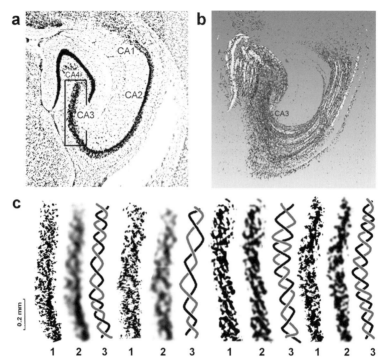

Fig 12.7   (a) A section through the Nissl-stained hippocampus of a gerbil suggests that helical structures may be hidden in the so-called 'hippocampus proper' or Ammon's horn, especially in the part called CA3. Each single dot corresponds to a neuron. (b) A 3D reconstruction of a series of Nissl-stained sections through the same structure reveals the curly appearance of the thin and bended Ammon's horn. (c) Four Nissl-stained sections through CA3 at different locations. The blurred images and the corresponding graphic interpretations suggest a double-helical structure that contains at least five turns (brain sections from http://en.wikipedia.org/wiki/Hippocampus).

The seemingly helical organization of a central part of the HC supports the view that the frequency of brain waves must be important for the activation of memory networks as well as for the storage and retrieval of the corresponding memory contents. If a part of a network, which represents a specific aspect of memory content, is activated with the right frequency, the whole network should tend to synchronize with this frequency. This resonance might explain why only a small sensory hint could be sufficient to evoke a complex 'memory – just' as in the case of Proust, when the taste of a Madeleine soaked in tea evoked extensive memories of his childhood.

In line with the assumption that CA3 may contribute to the selection and amplification of memory-related oscillations, it was found to generate oscillations from delta to gamma frequencies (0.5–100 Hz). Moreover, the oscillations were shown to propagate to CA1 (Fisahn *et al.*, 1998; Fellous and Sejnowski, 2000) where – comparable to neurons in the auditory midbrain – different types of neurons have distinct frequency preferences and act as band-pass filters (Pike *et al.*, 2000). In addition, compelling evidence has been accumulated to indicate that memory consolidation or learning is improved by a replay of memory-related oscillations during sleep. For example, neurons in the song system of sleeping birds have been observed to repeat the rhythms of newly learned songs (Margoliash, 2005). Also, EEG recordings in humans have shown that hippocampus-dependent memories benefit especially from low frequencies during sleep (Born *et al.*, 2006).

On the other hand, the coordination of memory replays in songbirds, as well as in rats which have learned to orient in a maze (Jones and Wilson, 2005), seems to be mediated by high-frequency oscillations. The frequencies and phases of the corresponding 'sharp wave-ripples' (high-frequency oscillations) of 200 Hz were demonstrated to be under tight control of the hippocampus (Buszáki, 2006; Edelman, 2010).

12.3.5   The 'black' helix

Another important formation in our brain which seems to contain a helical structure is the substantia nigra. The name reflects its black appearance in Nissl-stained brain sections. This complex structure in the midbrain consists of two substructures; the pars compacta (SNc) and pars reticulata (SNr) and is, together with the striatum and the pallidum, part of the basal ganglia. The inputs of these nuclei originate from motor areas in the cortex and from the striatum, which also includes sensory and associative, memory-related activity. Neurons in these regions project their axons to various structures, such as the thalamus, the limbic system and the reticular formation.

The most important projection, which uses dopamine as a predominantly inhibitory transmitter, connects neurons in the SNc to the striatum. The major function of this connection seems to be the control of motor commands that reach the striatum from the cortex. This is in line with a model according to which the task of the basal ganglia is to select a particular motor programme while inhibiting competing ones (Mink, 2003). More generally, it was suggested that the basal ganglia support attentional mechanisms which bind input to output in the forebrain (Brown and Marsden, 1998; Singer, 2013).

In Nissl-stained sections both substructures of the substantia nigra sometimes appear partly helical, although this is more obvious for the SNc. An example of such a stained section from a human brain is shown in Fig. 12.8a. Naturally, the section contains only a small fraction of the complete structure but, again, side views of a 3D reconstruction based on 12 sections from the same structure suggest an underlying helical organization (Fig. 12.8b, c).

Finally, in the graphic interpretation of the 3D organization (Fig. 12.8d), the SNc is akin to a double helix with about three and a half turns.

The existence of a helix in the substantia nigra implies that its control of motor functions is achieved through the control of brain oscillations. Obvious malfunctions of this structure should therefore result in either a reduction or an increase of oscillation amplitudes and thereby of the corresponding motor actions.

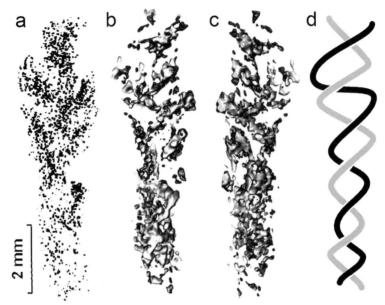

Fig 12.8   **(a)** A section from a Nissl-stained human brain that shows the distribution of cells in the substantia nigra, pars compacta (material courtesy of R. Galuske, MPI for Brain Research, Frankfurt). Bands of neurons are arranged in a way that suggests a 3D double-helical organization containing about three turns. **(b)** Lateral view of a 3D reconstruction based on 12 sections from the same brain. **(c)** The same reconstruction rotated by about 120 degrees. **(d)** The artistic interpretation of the 3D reconstruction suggests a double-helical organization with about three and a half turns.

A well-known syndrome that originates from malfunctioning of the substantia nigra is Parkinson's disease. A loss of neurons in the substantia nigra is the underlying cause of muscle stiffness and physical inactivity in Parkinson patients. In extreme cases patients may become nearly completely immobile, as was dramatically shown in the 1990 movie *Awakenings*. It is based on the memoirs of the famous neurologist Oliver Sacks, who successfully administered the drug L-Dopa, a precursor of dopamine, to his patients. As a consequence they were awakened – unfortunately for only a limited time – to a nearly normal life and could interact socially. The movie also demonstrated impressively how certain rhythmic stimuli, such as music or the periodicity of stairs, had unique effects on some patients, probably by enhancing or triggering brain oscillations.

At the other extreme, a malfunction of the basal ganglia characterized by a hyper-activity of its neurons probably results – in our interpretation – in uncontrollable or overemphasized brain oscillations leading to uncontrollable motor actions. This is the case in Huntington's chorea, Tourette's syndrome (with typical symptoms of mouth twitching or shouting of words) and obsessive-compulsive disorders (with symptoms such as excessive washing). For example, seeing a basin, such a patient would not be able to control or stop the elicited brain oscillation leading to an urge to wash his hands.

12.4   The mind is the 'music' of the brain

12.4.1   Periodicity analysis beyond the auditory system

The data presented in Figs. 12.4–12.8 suggest that helical-like anatomical structures exist not only in the auditory system (VNLL), but also in several non-auditory brain systems. While this may be just a peculiarity of brain anatomy and development without further functional significance, it seems more likely that their function is in some way comparable to that of the VNLL. This hypothesis leads to conclusions which can be tested for their plausibility. The most relevant conclusion may be that there should be correlation mechanisms for brain waves that are comparable to the auditory analysis of periodicity and the harmonic control of acoustically evoked oscillations. In the following paragraphs, a few additional topics will be addressed briefly. They indicate that periodicity analysis may indeed play a role in systems other than the auditory system and support the idea of György Buszáki that 'the rhythms of the brain are also the rhythms of the mind' (Buszáki, 2006).

12.4.2   Delay mechanisms and coincidence neurons

As we know from the model presented in Chapter 9, the analysis of periodicity first of all needs a well-defined delay (or delay difference) as a time reference. According to the model, the delays for the auditory periodicity analysis are mainly the result of processing in the dorsal cochlear nucleus (DCN). The comparatively small DCN is often called the cerebellum of the auditory system, because the spatial arrangement and connections of its neurons show a remarkable similarity to this large processing centre in the brain (see Fig. 7.11). The cerebellum is believed to function as a temporal processor or 'biological clock' (Braitenberg, 1983) characterized not only by delays but also by neuronal oscillations and coincidence detection. The delay lines are provided by billions of so-called granule cells, which send their long parallel axons through the large and flat dendritic trees of the Purkinje cells. These cells detect coincidences of spikes, probably mostly, but certainly not exclusively, for the control of motor actions. Furthermore, it was found that the cerebellum may oscillate over a frequency range extending from about 7 to 200 Hz. As a result, the Purkinje cells induce periodic inhibition in their target neurons of the deep cerebellar nuclei which, in consequence, tend to also oscillate in this range (Llinás and Mühlethaler, 1988; Loewenstein et al., 2005). Different frequencies are important for different functions. While high-frequency oscillations seem to support fast and precise movements, low frequencies are significant for interactions of the cerebellum with the sensorimotor cortex, supporting learning, arousal and attention (d'Angelo et al., 2009).

Another structure which may be involved in comparable temporal processing covering a large range of frequencies is the pallidum, a part of the basal ganglia (see Subsection 12.3.5; Buszáki, 2006). The anatomical organization of the pallidum is strikingly similar to the cerebellar architecture – even its major neurons resemble the Purkinje cells of the cerebellum with their extraordinary flat dendritic trees.

Temporal processing of oscillations requires precise coincidence detection as a decision-making device. Consequently, Purkinje cells in the cerebellum are by no means a rare example of coincidence detectors outside the auditory system. Actually, each neuron is sensitive to the coincidence of its inputs and the only questions that arise are how small or large its coincidence window and how precise its temporal response property is. For example, neurons in the cortex have a variety of specific functional features which make them highly sensitive coincidence detectors (Singer, 2007). Accordingly, they indicate precise timing of their inputs when oscillating with high frequencies, but there are also neurons that are involved in low-frequency oscillations and therefore are able to integrate longer time intervals.

12.4.3   The top-down control of oscillation frequency

Attention allows us to concentrate on or to select a neuronal oscillation which may represent, for example, a sound, a picture, a thought or an emotion (Başar et al., 2000). Obviously neuronal control centres are needed which support the selection or enhancement of behaviourally important oscillations and suppress other less important oscillations. For this purpose, the corresponding brain structures should somehow be able to recognize and address those neurons which are synchronized to an oscillation and thereby belong to a certain cell assembly.

It is difficult to imagine how the brain might manage to use the parameter of synchronization for this purpose. Indeed, it was argued that the theory of binding may be incomplete, or even untenable, because it describes synchronization as the signature of binding but does not detail how this synchronization could actually be computed in the brain (Shadlen and Movshon, 1999). For example, neurons which participate in an oscillation with a certain frequency could still differ significantly in synchronization strength or phase. Hence, it is an open but vital question as to how the brain would ever be able to address those neurons which are synchronized at a given moment and therefore belong to an activated neuronal ensemble.

A possible solution for this potentially serious flaw of the binding theory might be offered by exploiting the oscillation frequency. An advantage would be that even if the neurons which contribute to an oscillation were only weakly synchronized, appropriate correlation mechanisms could still determine their frequency. As in the auditory system, this would then allow the brain to engage appropriate inhibitory neurons which could enhance this oscillation by synchronized and properly timed inhibition while oscillations with other frequencies would be attenuated (see Fig. 11.6). Correspondingly, inhibition was found to be a key determinant of both synchronization and frequency of oscillations in other systems, for example in the hippocampus and the cortex (Bartos et al., 2007; Singer, 2013).

The usage of a certain frequency, instead of synchronization, for addressing the neurons of an assembly may be compared to the function of a broadcasting system (Glassman, 1999). Such a system does not need to know where its receivers are located but can still be sure that all those who are tuned in will receive the message. A control centre, for example the LC with its kilometres of axonal wiring, can 'broadcast' its message about the significance of certain oscillations over perhaps the whole cortex.

There is another advantage of using frequency as an essential control parameter. If a neuronal net is characterized by a certain oscillation frequency, the activation of only a small part of a neural net could possibly suffice to activate the whole net. In a way, memory recall may thus be considered as a kind of resonance effect. Stimulating the right cortical location with the right frequency will eventually activate the whole associated neural net because neurons at other locations will resonate. Finally, more or less large arrays of the cortex may be engaged, which possibly may represent comprehensive memory content. Perhaps this is what Marcel Proust found out when sipping his tea with cake evoked emotional feelings about his childhood, or stepping on a wobbly flagstone brought to mind old memories from Venice.

Note that the suggested mechanism for the selection of oscillation frequencies differs significantly from the 'winner-takes-all' principle which is well known in theoretical neuroscience. The idea of this principle is that a neuronal signal dominates just because it is stronger than other concurrent ones and therefore determines the progress of neuronal activation (mostly by inhibitory interactions). In contrast, the selection-by-frequency mode implies that by favouring a certain frequency superior brain centres may 'decide' and determine by top-down interference which oscillation should dominate. Corresponding top-down influences on gamma oscillations have been observed in visual memory tasks (Tallon-Baudry *et al.*, 1998).

12.4.4   A map for periodicity in the striatum?

It seems that the periodotopic organization in the auditory midbrain is essential for the representation of information contained in acoustic signals. As we have seen, it may be the spatial distribution of neuronal responses which allows us to recognize the pitches of acoustic signals as well as their harmonic relationships. The feedback of this information through the projections of neurons in the midbrain to the VNLL contributes to sharpness and selectivity of periodicity filtering, as required, for example, in cocktail parties.

To my knowledge nobody has ever raised the question of whether there are periodotopic maps elsewhere in the brain which may be important for the processing of EEG oscillations. The idea is that brain structures with topographic arrangements of periodicity-tuned neurons could be systematically employed to activate the neurons in corresponding helical structures, which then, by means of well-timed and synchronized inhibition, could enhance or attenuate particular brain oscillations. As a matter of fact there is evidence for some kind of a spatial representation of periodicity information in the striatum. This structure is the largest nucleus of the basal ganglia, with inputs from all regions of the cortex, the thalamus and the hippocampus. The evidence comes from a detailed analysis of gamma and theta oscillations recorded from multiple implanted electrodes in the striatum of rats. While gamma frequencies around 50 Hz were found to be strong in the ventro-medial region, theta frequencies around 7 Hz clearly dominated in the dorso-lateral region of the striatum (Berke *et al.*, 2004).

If the striatum does indeed contain a map for periodicity, one would expect that its neurons function like the neurons in the inferior colliculus as coincidence detectors. Indeed, a major task of the striatum seems to be to detect the temporal coincidence of its cortical inputs, which are characterized by phase delays between different oscillation frequencies. The delays may extend to seconds or even minutes and play an essential role for the exact timing of behaviour (Matell and Meck, 2004).

If one compares this processing with that of the periodicity processing in the auditory system, the cortex would play the role of the cochlear nucleus (CN), the striatum that of the auditory midbrain and the SN_c that of the VNLL. In the same way as delayed and undelayed CN signals coincide on neurons of the inferior colliculus, the phase-delayed cortical oscillations impinge on the 'spiny' coincidence neurons of the striatum. Moreover, just as neurons of the auditory midbrain innervate the VNLL, the coincidence neurons of the striatum activate the SN_c. Finally, similarly to the inhibition of the inferior colliculus by the VNLL, the SN_c provides dopaminergic inhibitory feedback to the striatum. It is in line with this comparison that this feedback 'provides a reinforcement signal to selectively weight cortical and thalamic inputs', just like the VNLL input does for the CN input to the auditory midbrain (Matell and Meck, 2004).

12.4.5   Neuronal space and harmony

As we know from acoustics, energy loss due to friction in air or water means that high frequencies fade more rapidly than low frequencies. This explains, for example, why low frequencies dominate in a thunderstorm and whales use infrasound for long-distance communication. Brain waves propagate in the cortex with speeds in the order of a few millimetres to several centimetres per second (Nunez and Shrinivasan, 2006). Because the length of waves (λ) is proportional to their speed (v) and inversely related to their frequency (f; $\lambda = v/f$), the maxima of gamma frequencies repeat in distances of millimetres or less and those of low frequencies do so in the centimetre range.

Therefore, high frequencies, like those in the gamma range, are well suited to synchronize closely neighbouring cortical locations, while low frequencies (in the alpha range or below) may synchronize locations that are more spatially separated. For example, while processing in the visual cortex is dominated by beta and gamma frequencies, multimodal semantic processing in neighbouring cortex areas favours alpha frequencies, and long-range interactions during memory tasks and mental imagery make use of the lower theta and delta frequencies (Stein and Sarnthein, 2000; Jensen et al., 2002). Accordingly, the synchronicity of gamma oscillations was repeatedly shown to fade away when the distance between recording sites was more than about 1 pcm (Eckhorn, 1994).

The fading of synchronicity, however, raises questions regarding the hypothesis that feature binding is mediated by coherent neuronal activity. After all, coherencies should not be restricted to locally stored features but should also be found between distant areas.

The necessary binding across long distances may not be possible without mediation of central hubs, such as the LC or substantia nigra, which – as their helical appearances suggest – may also involve the harmonic structure of ongoing oscillations (see below).

Probably, details of memory contents or other cognitive items are processed and stored in adjacent cortical locations, while unrelated or distantly related aspects are more separated. As a consequence, gamma frequencies are particularly important for the processing of details, for accurate cognitive and other actions. In contrast, long alpha wavelengths are suitable for less related features of the processed items, which are especially typical of creative or dreamlike brain processes.

Indeed, during sleep and dreaming, frequencies of brain waves are extremely low. This may explain why our dreams often seem weird – things are bound together which are normally regarded as distant and unrelated while we are awake. On the other hand, unexpected associations, creativity and sometimes even new discoveries are characteristic for dreams and other relaxed states of mind. Perhaps a creative mind has the ability to effectively wander between low- and high-frequency processing, thereby combining surprising associations with a skilled handling of detailed information.

12.4.6   'Is grandmother a frequency composition?'

By now it should be clear why the original hypothesis of a 'grandmother cell' (see above) has been replaced in the last decades by the concept of a synchronized 'grandmother network'. This motivated the neuroscientist Stryker (1989) to ask the question: Is grandmother an oscillation?

It was a true inspiration, therefore, to investigate brain oscillations triggered by photos of real grandmothers (Başar et al., 2004). The resulting EEG measurements in these subjects showed that the superimposed oscillations elicited in this way are not only distributed over various brain areas but also through different frequency bands with varying degrees of amplitude, duration and delay. As Fig. 12.9 shows, alpha waves are dominant in the occipital pole of the brain, which is responsible for primary visual processing, while theta waves are dominant in the frontal cortex and are probably related to cognition and face recognition. It would certainly make sense, therefore, to change Stryker's question into: Is grandmother a frequency composition?

Certainly, these different brain waves which extend over several octaves have to be coordinated in some way, an aspect which was perhaps captured more closely in Carl Stumpf's old concept of fusion than in the newer binding principle, which is focused on neuronal nets oscillating with the same frequency. Anyhow, the conclusion seems unavoidable: if different frequencies in different brain areas contribute to a cognitive item, such as the memory of a grandmother, harmonic relations and harmonic interactions may be important for binding or fusion.

As we have seen in Chapter 11, harmonic relations of frequency do have an impact on periodicity coding in the auditory system. If a tone activates a coincidence neuron because its period matches the correlational delay provided by another input, then a

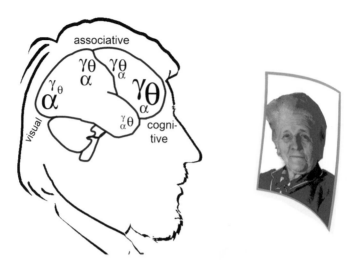

Fig. 12.9   The figure gives an artistic account of selectively distributed oscillations measured in different brain regions of subjects while facing images of their grandmother. The size of the Greek letters indicates the amplitude of the corresponding EEG waves in different brain regions (inspired by Başar *et al.*, 2004).

harmonically related tone may also be appropriate to activate this neuron. Similarly, if the neurons which are synchronized to a particular brain wave coincide on another neuron somewhere downstream, they do not necessarily have to fire in a 1:1 relationship in order to activate this neuron. Other harmonic ratios (2:1, 3:1, 3:2, etc.) may also be sufficient (Singer, 2007). Different combinations of frequencies may therefore have the same, or similar, effects on neurons in subsequent processing centres. Therefore, as for auditory processing, harmonic relationships must be an important aspect for the control and selection of oscillations and may depend on appropriate neuronal mechanisms.

The effect of this control may become more plausible by the following example: it is often said that people tend to be either 'splitters' or 'lumpers', seeing mostly either trees or woods. In the light of our oscillation theory, splitters should use preferentially higher and lumpers lower brain frequencies (see above). Since both processing modes have advantages and disadvantages, it would be certainly best to change frequencies in a controlled way. Moreover, since harmonically related frequencies should have similar effects downstream, it should be quite efficient to switch not arbitrarily but between harmonically related frequencies. Such a harmonic control should be possible by means of helical control centres that allow our mind to wander, for example from one thought to another related one or from perceptual details to associations. Thinking would be comparable to the humming of a melody or the playing of a musical instrument – or as Robert Glassman wrote (1999): 'If there is indeed a brain wave frequency code for cognitive item-representations ... the simple mathematical relationships of harmonies could provide a basis for maintaining distinctness and orderly changes. Thus, a basic aspect of music may provide a model for an essential characteristic of working memory.'

In conclusion, we could imagine our brain as a musical instrument or, perhaps better, as a whole orchestra. The instruments would then be the neuronal nets distributed all over the cortex and there would be all kinds of such instruments – small and large, loud or soft, of high or low pitch. To a certain extent we may be listeners, musicians or, under optimal conditions, even the conductor of this orchestra. More so than with acoustic music, it would certainly be of importance which instruments are playing at a certain time and also where they are located. Finally, certainly in line with those of Pythagoras as discussed in Chapter 1, these philosophical speculations may possibly culminate in the somewhat esoteric thesis that 'our mind is the music of the brain'.

Perhaps the best summary for the present chapter comes from the introduction of a paper from Başar and co-authors (2001). They wrote:

A great change has taken place in Neuroscience. Brain scientists have recognized the importance of oscillatory phenomena and the functional EEG. This new development will not only govern improvements in Neuroscience within the next two or three decades, it will probably create the basic approach for the biophysical understanding of brain machinery.

References

Adams, J. C. 1983. Multipolar cells in the ventral cochlear nucleus project to the dorsal cochlear nucleus and the inferior colliculus. *Neuroscience Letters* 37: 205–208.

Adams, J. C. 1997. Projections from octopus cells of the posteroventral cochlear nucleus to the ventral nucleus of the lateral lemniscus in cat and human. *Auditory Neuroscience* 3: 335–350.

Ade, P. A., Aikin, R. W., Barkats, D., *et al.* 2014. BICEP2 I: detection of B-mode polarization at degree angular scales. *Physical Review Letters* 112, doi: http://dx.doi.org/10.1103/PhysRevLett.112.241101.

Aertsen, A. M. H. J. and Johannesma, P. I. M. 1980. Spectro-temporal receptive fields in auditory neurons in the grassfrog: I. Characterization of tonal and natural stimuli. *Biological Cybernetics* 38(4): 223–234.

Aggleton, J. P. 1993. The contribution of the amygdala to normal and abnormal emotional states. *Trends in Neuroscience* 16(8): 328–333.

Albert, M. 1994. Verarbeitung komplexer akustischer Signale im Colliculus inferior des Chinchillas: Funktionelle Eigenschaft und topographische Repräsentation. PhD diss., Darmstadt, TU-Darmstadt.

Aston-Jones, G. and Cohen, J. D. 2005. An integrative theory of locus coeruleus–norepinephrine function: adaptive gain and optimal performance. *Annual Reviews in Neuroscience* 28(1): 403–450.

Bachem, A. 1955. Absolute pitch. *Journal of the Acoustical Society of America* 27: 1180–1185.

Bahmer, A. and Langner, G. 2006a. Oscillating neurons in the cochlear nucleus: I. Experimental basis of a simulation paradigm. *Biological Cybernetics* 95: 371–379.

Bahmer, A. and Langner, G. 2006b. Oscillating neurons in the cochlear nucleus: II. Simulation results. *Biological Cybernetics* 95(4): 381–392.

Bahmer, A. and Langner, G. 2007. Simulation of oscillating neurons in the cochlear nucleus: a possible role for neural nets, onset cells, and synaptic delays. In Kollmeier, B., Klump, G., Langmann, U., *et al.* (eds), *Hearing: From Sensory Processing to Perception*. Berlin, Heidelberg: Springer: 155–164.

Bahmer, A. and Langner, G. 2009. A simulation of chopper neurons in the cochlear nucleus with wideband input from onset neurons. *Biological Cybernetics* 100(1): 21–33.

Barker, A. D. 2012. *The Oxford Classical Dictionary.* New York: Oxford University Press.

Barnea, A., Granot, R. and Pratt, H. 1994. Absolute pitch: electrophysiological evidence. *International Journal of Psychophysiology* 16(1): 29–38.

Bartos, M., Vida, I. and Jonas, P. 2007. Synaptic mechanisms of synchronized gamma oscillations in inhibitory interneuron networks. *Nature Reviews Neuroscience* 8(1): 45–56.

Başar, E., Başar-Eroğlu, C., Karakaş, S. and Schürmann, M. 2000. Brain oscillations in perception and memory. *International Journal of Psychophysiology* 35: 95–124.

Başar, E., Başar-Eroğlu, C., Karakaş, S. and Schürmann, M. 2001. Gamma, alpha, delta, and theta oscillations govern cognitive processes. *International Journal of Psychophysiology* 39: 241–248.

Başar, E., Başar-Eroğlu, C., Karakaş, S., Schürmann, M. and Ozgoron, M. 2004. Super-synergy in brain oscillations and the grandmother percept. *International Journal of Bifurcation and Chaos* 14: 453–491.

Batra, R. 2006. Responses of neurons in the ventral nucleus of the lateral lemniscus to sinusoidally amplitude modulated tones. *Journal of Neurophysiology* 96(5): 2388–2398.

Baumann S., Griffiths, T., Sun, L., *et al.* 2011. Orthogonal representation of sound dimensions in the primate midbrain. *Nature Neuroscience* 14(4): 423–425.

Bennett, M., Schatz, M., Rockwood, H. and Wiesenfeld, K. 2002. Huygens's clocks. *Proceedings: Mathematical, Physical and Engineering Sciences* 458: 563–579.

Benson, C. G. and Cant, N. B. 2008. The ventral nucleus of the lateral lemniscus of the gerbil (*Meriones unguiculatus*): organization of connections with the cochlear nucleus and the inferior colliculus. *Journal of Comparative Neurology* 510: 673–690.

Berke, J. D., Okatan, M., Skurski, J. and Eichenbaum, H. B. 2004. Oscillatory entrainment of striatal neurons in freely moving rats. *Neuron* 43(6): 883–896.

Bernstein, J. G. and Oxenham, A. J. 2003. Pitch discrimination of diotic and dichotic tone complexes: harmonic resolvability or harmonic number? *Journal of the Acoustical Society of America* 113: 3323–3334.

Bibikov, N. G. 1974. Encoding of the stimulus envelope in peripheral and central regions of the auditory system of the frog. *Acta Acoustica* 31: 310–314.

Bibikov, N. G. and Nizamov, S. V. 1996. Temporal coding of low-frequency amplitude modulation in the torus semicircularis of the grass frog. *Hearing Research* 101(1): 23–44.

Bidelman, G. M. and Krishnan, A. 2009. Neural correlates of consonance, dissonance, and the hierarchy of musical pitch in the human brainstem. *Journal of Neuroscience* 21: 13165–13171.

Biebel, U. W. and Langner, G. 2002. Evidence for interactions across frequency channels in the inferior colliculus of awake chinchilla. *Hearing Research* 169: 151–168.

Birch, T. 1757. *The History of the Royal Society of London for Improving of Natural Knowledge, From Its First Rise: In Which the Most Considerable of Those Papers Communicated to the Society, Which Have Hitherto not Been Published, are Inserted in their Proper Order, as a Supplement to the Philosophical Transactions* (Vol. 3). London: A. Millar.

Bishop, P. O. 1953. Synaptic transmission: an analysis of the electrical activity of the lateral geniculate nucleus in the cat after optic nerve stimulation. *Proceedings of the Royal Society B: Biological Sciences* 141: 362–392.

Blackburn, C. C. and Sachs, M. B. 1989. Classification of unit types in the anteroventral cochlear nucleus: PST histograms and regularity analysis. *Journal of Neurophysiology* 62: 1303–1329.

Bodnar, D. A. and Bass, A. H. 2001. Coding of concurrent vocal signals by the auditory midbrain: effects of stimulus level and depth of modulation. *Journal of the Acoustical Society of America* 109: 809–825.

Boethius, A. M. S. 1989. *Fundamentals of Music.* Translated by C. M. Bower, New Haven, CT and London: Yale University Press.

Bonke, D., Scheich, H. and Langner, G. 1979. Responsiveness of units in the auditory neostriatum of the guinea fowl (*Numida meleagris*) to species-specific calls and synthetic stimuli. *Journal of Comparative Physiology* 132: 243–255.

Born, J. A. N. and Wagner, U. 2004. Memory consolidation during sleep: role of cortisol feedback. *Annals of the New York Academy of Sciences* 1032: 198–201.

Born, J., Rasch, B. R. and Gais, S. 2006. Sleep to remember. *Neuroscience* 12: 410–424.

Borst, J. G. G., Helmchen, F. and Sakmann, B. 1995. Pre- and postsynaptic whole-cell recordings in the medial nucleus of the trapezoid body of the rat. *Journal of Physiology* 489(3): 825–840.

Borst, M., Palm, G. and Langner, G. 2004. A biologically motivated neural network for phase extraction from complex sounds. *Biological Cybernetics* 90: 98–104.

Bourk, T. R. 1976. Electrical responses of neural units in the antero-ventral cochlear nucleus of the cat. PhD diss., MIT, Cambridge, MA.

Braitenberg, V. 1983. The cerebellum revisited. *Journal of Theoretical Neurobiology* 2: 237–241.

Britt, R. and Starr, A. 1976. Synaptic events and discharge patterns of cochlear nucleus cells: I. Steady-frequency tone bursts. *Journal of Neurophysiology* 39: 162–178.

Brosch, M., Budinger, E. and Scheich, H. 2002. Stimulus-related gamma oscillations in primate auditory cortex. *Journal of Neurophysiology* 87: 2715–2725.

Brown, P. and Marsden, C. D. 1998. What do the basal ganglia do? *The Lancet* 351: 1801–1804.

Brugge, J. F. Blatchley, B. and Kudoh, M. 1993. Encoding of amplitude-modulated tones by neurons of the inferior colliculus of the kitten. *Brain Research* 615: 199–217.

Bullock, T. H. 1961. The problem of recognition in an analyzer made of neurons. In Rosenblith, W. A. (ed.), *Sensory Communication*. Cambridge, MA: Technical Press: 717–724.

Burger, R. M. and Pollak, G. D. 1998. Analysis of the role of inhibition in shaping responses to sinusoidally amplitude-modulated signals in the inferior colliculus. *Journal of Neurophysiology* 80: 1686–1701.

Burns, E. M. and Campbell, S. L. 1994. Frequency and frequency-ratio resolution by possessors of absolute and relative pitch: examples of categorical perception? *Journal of the Acoustical Society of America* 96(5): 2704–2719.

Buzsáki, G. 2006. *Rhythms of the Brain*. New York: Oxford University Press.

Cant, N. B. and Benson, C. G. 2003. Parallel auditory pathways: projection patterns of the different neuronal populations in the dorsal and ventral cochlear nuclei. *Brain Research Bulletin* 60: 457–474.

Cant, N. B. and Benson, C. G. 2008. Organization of the inferior colliculus of the gerbil (*Meriones unguiculatus*): projections from the cochlear nucleus. *Neuroscience* 154: 206–217.

Caspary, D. M., Rupert, A. L. and Moushegian, G. 1977. Neuronal coding of vowel sounds in the cochlear nuclei. *Experimental Neurology* 54: 414–431.

Caspary, D. M., Palombi, P. S. and Hughes, L. F. 2002. GABAergic inputs shape responses to amplitude modulated stimuli in the inferior colliculus. *Hearing Research* 168: 163–173.

Cetas, J. S., Price, R. O., Velenovsky, D. S., Sinex, D. G. and McMullen, N. T. 2001. Frequency organization and cellular lamination in the medial geniculate body of the rabbit. *Hearing Research* 155: 113–123.

Chistovich, L. A. and Lublinskaya, V. V. 1979. The center of gravity effect in vowel spectra and critical distance between the formants: psychoacoustical study of the perception of vowel-like stimuli. *Hearing Research* 1: 185–195.

Chung, D. Y. and Colavita, F. B. 1976. Periodicity pitch perception and its upper frequency limit in cats. *Perception and Psychophysics* 20: 433–437.

Chung, D. Y. and Geissmann, T. 2000. Gibbon songs and human music from an evolutionary perspective. In Wallin, N. L., Merker, B. and Brown, S. (eds), *The Origins of Music*. Cambridge, MA: MIT Press: 103–123.

Clodoré-Tissot, T. 2009. *Instruments sonorés du Néolithique à l'aube de l'Antiquité*. Cahier XII, Paris: Éditions S. P. F.

Conard, N. J., Malina, M. and Münzel, S. C. 2009. New flutes document the earliest musical tradition in southwestern Germany. *Nature* 460: 737–740.

Condon, C. J., White, K. R. and Feng, A. S. 1996. Neurons with different temporal firing patterns in the inferior colliculus of the little brown bat differentially process sinusoidal amplitude-modulated signals. *Journal of Comparative Physiology A: Sensory, Neural and Behavioral Physiology* 178: 147–157.

Covey, E. and Casseday, J. H. 1999. Timing in the auditory system of the bat. *Annual Review of Physiology* 61(1): 457–476.

Covey, E., Kauer, J. A. and Casseday, J. H. 1996. Whole-cell patch-clamp recording reveals subthreshold sound-evoked postsynaptic currents in the inferior colliculus of awake bats. *Journal of Neuroscience* 16: 3009–3018.

Cynx, J. and Shapiro, M. 1986. Perception of missing fundamental by a species of songbird (*Sturnus vulgaris*). *Journal of Comparative Psychology* 100: 356–360.

d'Angelo, E., Koekkoek, S., Lombardo, P., *et al.* 2009. Timing in the cerebellum: oscillations and resonance in the granular layer. *Journal of Neuroscience* 162: 805–815.

Darwin, C. 2004. *The Descent of Man*. Digireads.com Publishing.

Dau, T., Kollmeier, B. and Kohlrausch, B. 1997. Modeling auditory processing of amplitude modulation: II. Spectral and temporal integration. *Journal of the Acoustical Society of America* 102: 2906–2919.

de Boer, E. 1956. Pitch of inharmonic signals. *Nature* 178: 535–536.

de Cheveigne, A. 2005. Pitch perception models. In Plack, C. J., Fay, R. R., Oxenham, A. J. and Poppe, A.N. (eds), *Pitch. Neural Coding and Perception*. New York: Springer: 169–233.

Decker, J. 1986. Simulation eines neuronalen Korrelationsmodells für eine akustische Periodenanalyse. Thesis, Darmstadt: TU-Darmstadt.

Delgutte, B. 1980. Representation of speech-like sounds in the discharge patterns of auditory nerve fibers. *Journal of the Acoustical Society of America* 68: 843–857.

Delgutte, B. and Kiang, N. Y. 1984. Speech coding in the auditory nerve: I. Vowel-like sounds. *Journal of the Acoustical Society of America* 75: 866–878.

Dermott, S. F. 1973. Bode's law and the resonant structure of the solar system. *Nature Physical Science* 244: 18–21.

Deutsch, D., Henthorn, T., Marvin, E. and Xu, H. 2006. Absolute pitch among American and Chinese conservatory students: prevalence differences, and evidence for a speech-related critical period. *Journal of the Acoustical Society of America* 119: 719–722.

Dinse, H. R., Godde, B., Hilger, T., *et al.* 1997. Optical imaging of cat auditory cortex cochleotopic selectivity evoked by acute electrical stimulation of a multi-channel cochlear implant. *European Journal of Neuroscience* 9: 113–119.

Drobisch, M. W. 1855. *Über musikalische Tonbestimmug und Temperatur*. Abhandlungen der Mathematisch-Physkalischen Classe der Königlich-Sächsischen Gesellschaft der Wissenschaften zu Leipzig (www.uni-leipzig).

Ebeling, M. 2008. Neuronal periodicity detection as a basis for the perception of consonance: a mathematical model of tonal fusion. *Journal of the Acoustical Society of America* 124: 2320–2329.

Eccles, J. C. 1964. *The Physiology of Synapses*. Berlin: Springer.

Eckhorn, R. 1994. Oscillatory and non-oscillatory synchronizations in the visual cortex and their possible roles in the associations of visual features. *Progress in Brain Research* 102: 405–426.

Eckhorn, R., Bauer, R., Jordan, W., *et al.* 1988. Coherent oscillations: a mechanism of feature linking in the visual cortex? *Biological Cybernetics* 60: 121–130.

Edelman, S. 2010. On look-ahead in language: navigating a multitude of familiar paths. In Bar, M. (ed.), *Prediction in the Brain: Using the Past to Generate the Future.* New York: Oxford University Press: 170–189.

Egorova, M. and Ehret, G. 2008. Tonotopy and inhibition in the midbrain inferior colliculus shape spectral resolution of sounds in neural critical bands. *European Journal of Neuroscience* 28(4): 675–692.

Eguia, M. C., Garcia, G. C. and Romano, S. A. 2010. A biophysical model for modulation frequency encoding in the cochlear nucleus. *Journal of Physiology* 104: 118–127.

Ehret, G. 1997. The auditory cortex. *Journal of Comparative Physiology A* 181:547–557.

Ehret, G. and Merzenich, M. M. 1985. Auditory midbrain responses parallel spectral integration phenomena. *Science* 227: 1245–1247.

Engel, A. K. and Singer, W. 2001. Temporal binding and the neural correlates of sensory awareness. *Trends in Cognitive Sciences* 5: 16–25.

Epping, W. J. M. and Eggermont, J. J. 1986. Sensitivity of neurons in the auditory midbrain of the grassfrog to temporal characteristics of sound: II. Stimulation with amplitude modulated sounds. *Hearing Research* 24: 55–72.

Evans, E. F. and Nelson, P. G. 1973. The responses of single neurons in the cochlear nucleus of the cat as a function of their location and the anaesthetic state. *Experimental Brain Research* 17: 402–427.

Evans, E. and Palmer, A. 1980. Relationship between the dynamic range of cochlear nerve fibres and their spontaneous activity. *Experimental Brain Research* 40: 115–118.

Faingold, C. L., Gehlbach, G. and Caspary, D. M. 1989. On the role of GABA as an inhibitory neurotransmitter in inferior colliculus neurons: iontophoretic studies. *Brain Research* 500: 301–312.

Fellous, J. M. and Sejnowski, T. J. 2000. Cholinergic induction of oscillations in the hippocampal slice in the slow (0.5–2 Hz), theta (5–12 Hz), and gamma (35–70 Hz) bands. *Hippocampus* 10: 187–197.

Ferragamo, M. J., Golding, N. L. and Oertel, D. 1998. Synaptic inputs to stellate cells in the ventral cochlear nucleus. *Journal of Neurophysiology* 79: 51–63.

Fisahn, A., Pike, F. G., Buhl, E. H. and Paulsen, O. 1998. Cholinergic induction of network oscillations at 40 Hz in the hippocampus in vitro. *Nature* 394: 186–189.

Fishman, Y. I., Volkov, I. O., Noh, M. D., *et al.* 2001. Consonance and dissonance of musical chords: neural correlates in auditory cortex of monkeys and humans. *Journal of Neurophysiology* 86(6): 2761–2788.

Fletcher, H. and Munson, W. A. 1933. Loudness, its definition, measurements and calculation. *Journal of the Acoustical Society of America* 5: 82–108.

Fourier, J. B. J. 1822. *Théorie analytique de la chaleur.* Didot.

Fries, P. 2009. Neuronal gamma-band synchronisation as a fundamental process in cortical computation. *Annual Review of Neuroscience* 32: 209–224.

Fries, P., Reynold, J., Rorie, A. and Desimone, R. 2001. Modulation of oscillatory neuronal synchronisation by selective visual attention. *Science* 291(5508): 1560–1563.

Frisina, R. D., Walton, J. P., Lynch-Armour, M. A., Hackett, J. T., Jackson, H. and Rubel, E. W. 1982. Synaptic excitation of the second and third order auditory neurons in the avian brain stem. *Neuroscience* 7: 1455–1469.

Frisina, R. D., Smith, R. L. and Chamberlain. S. C. 1985. Differential encoding of rapid changes in sound amplitude by second order auditory neurons. *Experimental Brain Research* 60: 417–422.

Frisina, R. D., Smith, R. L. and Chamberlain, S. C. 1990. Encoding of amplitude modulation in the gerbil cochlear nucleus: II. Possible neural mechanisms. *Hearing Research* 44: 123–142.

Frisina, R. D., Walton, J. P. and Karcich, K. J. 1994. Dorsal cochlear nucleus single neurons can enhance temporal processing capabilities in background noise. *Experimental Brain Research* 102(1): 160–164.

Frisina, R. D., Wang, J., Byrd, J., *et al.* 1997. Enhanced processing of temporal features of sounds in background noise by cochlear nucleus single neurons. In Syka, J. (ed.), *Acoustical Signal Processing in the Central Auditory System*. New York: Plenum Press: 109–125.

Fritz, T., Jentschke, S., Gosselin, N., *et al.* 2009. Universal recognition of three basic emotions in music. *Current Biology* 19: 573–576.

Gabrielsson, A. 2012. *Strong Experiences with Music: Music is Much More Than Just Music.* Oxford: Oxford Scholarship.

Gaffurius, F. 1492.*Theorica musice*. Edited by Illuminati, I. and Bellissima, F. Firenze: Edizioni del Galluzzo (2005).

Geissmann, T. 2002. Duet-splitting and the evolution of gibbon songs. *Biological Reviews* 77(1): 57–76.

Gibson, G., Warren, B. and Russell, I. J. 2010. Humming in tune: sex and species recognition by mosquitoes on the wing. *Journal of the Association for Research in Otolaryngology* 11(4): 527–540.

Glassman, R. B. 1999. Hypothesized neural dynamics of working memory: several chunks might be marked simultaneously by harmonic frequencies within an octave band of brain waves. *Brain Research Bulletin* 50(2): 77–93.

Glattke, T. J. 1969. Unit responses of the cat cochlear nucleus to amplitude-modulated stimuli. *Journal of the Acoustical Society of America* 45: 419–425.

Godfrey, D. A., Kiang, N. Y. S. and Norris, B. E. 1975. Single unit activity in the posteroventral cochlear nucleus of the cat. *Journal of Comparative Neurology* 162: 247–268.

Goldberg, J. M. and Brownell, W. E. 1973. Discharge characteristics of neurons in anteroventral and dorsal cochlear nuclei of cat. *Brain Research* 64: 35–54.

Goldstein, J. L. 1973. An optimum processor theory for the central formation of the pitch of complex tones. *Journal of the Acoustical Society of America* 54: 1496–1516.

Grace, A. A. 1991. Phasic versus tonic dopamine release and the modulation of dopamine system responsivity: a hypothesis for the etiology of schizophrenia. *Neuroscience* 41: 1–24.

Gray, C. M. 1999. The temporal correlation hypothesis of visual feature integration: still alive and well. *Neuron* 24: 31–47.

Gray, C. M., Engel, A. K., König, P. and Singer, W. 1990. Stimulus-dependent neuronal oscillations in cat visual cortex: inter-columnar interaction as determined by cross-correlation analysis. *European Journal of Neuroscience* 2(7): 607–619.

Greenberg, S. 1988. The ear as a speech analyzer. *Journal of Phonetics* 16: 139–149.

Griffiths, T. D. and Hall, D. A. 2012. Mapping pitch representation in neural ensembles with fMRI. *Journal of Neuroscience* 32(39): 13343–13347.

Griffiths, T. D. Büchel, C., Frackowiak, R. S. and Patterson, R. D. 1998. Analysis of temporal structure in sound by the human brain. *Nature Neuroscience* 1(5): 422–427.

Grinvald, A., Lieke, E., Frostig, R. D., Gilbert, C. D. and Wiesel, T. N. 1986. Functional architecture of cortex revealed by optical imaging of intrinsic signals. *Nature* 324: 361–364.

Gross, C. G. 2002. Genealogy of the 'grandmother cell'. *The Neuroscientist* 8(5): 512–518.

Gumbel, E. J., Greenwood, J. A. and Durand, D. 1953. The circular normal distribution: theory and tables. *Journal of the American Statistical Association* 48(261): 131–152.

Hahn, J. and Münzel, S. 1995. Knochenflöten aus dem Aurignacien des Geissenklösterle bei Blaubeuren. *Fundberichte aus Baden-Würtemberg* 20: 1–12.

Hall, D. A. and Plack, C. J. 2009. Pitch processing sites in the human auditory brain. *Cerebral Cortex* 19(3): 576–585.

Hartmann, W. M. 1997. *Sounds, Signals, and Sensation: Modern Acoustics and Signal Processing.* New York: Springer Verlag.

Hattori, T. and Suga, N. 1997. The inferior colliculus of the mustached bat has the frequency-vs-latency coordinates. *Journal of Comparative Physiology A* 180(3): 271–284.

Hebb, D. O. 1961. Distinctive features of learning in the higher animal. In Delafresnaye, J. F. (ed.), *Brain Mechanisms and Learning.* Oxford: Blackwell: 37–51.

Heffner, H. E. and Whitfield, I. C. 1976. Perception of the missing fundamental by cats. *Journal of the Acoustical Society of America* 59: 915–919.

Heil, P., Schulze, H. and Langner, G. 1995. Ontogenetic development of periodicity coding in the inferior colliculus of the mongolian gerbil. *Auditory Neuroscience* 1: 363–383.

Helmholtz, H. L. F. von 1863. *Die Lehre von den Tonempfindungen.* F. Vieweg und Sohn.

Helmholtz, H. L. F. von 1954. *On the Sensation of Tone.* New York: Dover Publications.

Hewitt, M. J., Meddis, R. and Shacklet, T. M. 1992. A computer-model of a cochlear-nucleus stellate cell: responses to amplitude-modulated and pure-tone stimuli. *Journal of the Acoustical Society of America* 91: 2096–2109.

Hickmann, E. 2007. *Klänge Altamerikas.* Darmstadt: Wissenschaftliche Buchgemeinschaft.

Hirsch, H. R. and Gibson, M. M. 1976. Responses of single units in the cat cochlear nucleus to sinusoidal amplitude modulation of tones and noise: linearity and relation to speech perception. *Journal of Neuroscience Research* 2: 337–356,

Hochmair, I. J. and Hochmair, E. S. 1986. *System for Enhancing Auditory Stimulation and the Like.* US Patent No. 4,577,641. Washington, DC: US Patent and Trademark Office.

Hopkins, C. D. 1974. Electric communication in the reproductive behavior of *Sternopygus macrurus* (Gymnotoidei). *Zeitschrift für Tierpsychologie* 35: 518–535.

Hornbostel, E. M. V. 1928. *Die Maßnorm als kulturgeschichtliches Forschungsmittel.* In Koppers, W. (ed.), *Festschrift.* Wien: Mechitharisten-Congregations-Buchdruckerei: 303–321.

Horst, J. W., Javel, E. and Farley, G. R. 1985. Extraction and enhancement of spectral structure by the cochlea. *Journal of the Acoustical Society of America* 78: 1898–1901.

Horst, J. W., Javel, E. and Farley, G. R. 1986. Coding of spectral fine-structure in the auditory-nerve: I. Fourier analysis of period and interspike interval histograms. *Journal of the Acoustical Society of America* 79: 398–416.

Horst, J. W., Javel, E. and Farley, G. R. 1990. Coding of spectral fine-structure in the auditory nerve: II. Level-dependent nonlinear responses. *Journal of the Acoustical Society of America* 88: 2656–2681.

Hose, B., Langner, G. and Scheich, H. 1983. Linear phoneme boundaries for German synthetic two-formant vowels. *Hearing Research* 9(1): 13–25.

Hose., B., Langner, G. and Scheich, H. 1987. Topographic representation of periodicities in the forebrain of the mynah bird: one map for pitch and rhythm? *Brain Research* 422: 367–373.

Hu, W. and White, M. 2004. The cosmic symphony. *Scientific American* 290(2): 44.

Hübner, R. 1997. The effect of spatial frequency on global precedence and hemispheric differences. *Perception & Psychophysics* 59: 187–201.

Hudspeth, A. J. 1997. Mechanical amplification of stimuli by hair cells. *Current Opinion in Neurobiology* 7: 480–486.

Huffman, R. F. and Covey, E. 1995. Origin of ascending projections to the nuclei of the lateral lemniscus in the big brown bat, *Eptesicus fuscus*. *Journal of Comparative Neurology* 357: 532–545.

Hulse, S. H. and Cynx, J. 1985. Relative pitch perception is constrained by absolute pitch in songbirds (*Mimus, Molothrus* and *Sturnus*). *Journal of Comparative Psychology* 99(2): 176–196.

Huxley, T. H. 1880. *The Crayfish: An Introduction to Zoology*. London: C. Kegan Paul & Co.

Jähn-Siebert, T. K. and Langner, G. 1995. Afferent innervation and intrinsic connections of isofrequency sheets in the central nucleus colliculus (icc) in the chinchilla: a double retrograd tracer study. *Learning and Memory* V: 318.

Javel, E. 1980. Coding of AM tones in the chinchilla auditory nerve: implications for the pitch of complex tones. *Journal of the Acoustical Society of America* 68: 133–146.

Javel, E. 1986. Basic response properties of auditory nerve fibers. In Altschuler, R. A, Hoffman, D. W. and Bobbin, R. P. (eds), *Neurobiology of Hearing: The Cochlea*. New York: Raven Press: 213–245.

Jeffress, L. A. 1948. A place theory of sound localization. *Journal of Comparative and Physiological Psychology* 41(1): 35–39.

Jensen, O., Gelfand, J., Kounios, J. and Lisman, J. E. 2002. Oscillations in the alpha band (9–12 Hz) increase with memory load during retention in a short-term memory task. *Cerebral Cortex* 12(8): 877–882.

Jones, M. W. and Wilson, M. A. 2005. Theta rhythms coordinate hippocampal–prefrontal interactions in a spatial memory task. *Public Library of Science Biology* 3: e402.

Joris, P. X. and. Smith, P. H. 1998. Temporal and binaural properties in dorsal cochlear nucleus and its output tract. *Journal of Neuroscience* 18: 10157–10170.

Joris, P. X. and Yin, T. C. T. 1992. Responses to amplitude-modulated tones in the auditory-nerve of the cat. *Journal of the Acoustical Society of America* 91: 215–232.

Kaernbach, C. and Bering, C. 2001. Exploring the temporal mechanism involved in the pitch of unresolved harmonics. *Journal of the Acoustical Society of America* 110: 1039–1048.

Kavanagh, J. F., Moore, J. K. and Osen, K. 1979. The cochlear nuclei in man. *American Journal of Anatomy* 154: 393–417.

Kazdin, A. 1989. *Glenn Could at Work: Creative Lying*. New York: E. P. Dutton.

Kim, D. O. and Molnar, C. E. 1979. A population study of cochlear nerve fibers: comparison of spatial distributions of average-rate and phase-locking measures of responses to single tones. *Journal of Neurophysiology* 42: 16–30.

Kim, D. O., Sirianni, J. G. and Chang, S. O. 1990. Responses of DCN-PVCN neurons and auditory nerve fibers in unanesthetized decerebrate cats to AM and pure tones: analysis with autocorrelation/power-spectrum. *Hearing Research* 45: 95–113.

Kimura, A., Imbe, H., Donishi, T. and Tamai, Y. 2007. Axonal projections of single auditory neurons in the thalamic reticular nucleus: implications for tonotopy-related gating function and cross-modal modulation. *European Journal of Neuroscience* 26: 3524–3535.

Klumpp, R. G. and Eady, H. R. 1956. Some measurements of interaural time difference thresholds. *Journal of the Acoustical Society of America* 28: 859–860.

Koelsch, S., Gunter, T., Friederici, A. D. and Schröger, E. 2000. Brain indices of music processing: nonmusicians are musical. *Journal of Cognitive Neuroscience* 12: 520–541.

Kraushaar, U. and Backus, K. H. 2002. Characterization of GABAA and glycine receptors in neurons of the developing rat inferior colliculus. *Pflügers Archiv* 445(2): 279–288.

Krishna, B. S. and Semple, M. N. 2000. Auditory temporal processing: responses to sinusoidally amplitude-modulated tones in the inferior colliculus. *Journal of Neurophysiology* 84: 255–273.

Krumbholz, K. Patterson, R. D., Seither-Preisler, A., Lammertmann, C. and Lütkenhöner, B. 2003. Neuromagnetic evidence for a pitch processing center in Heschl's gyrus. *Cerebral Cortex* 13(7): 765–772.

Krumhansl, C. L. 1990. *Cognitive Foundations of Musical Pitch*. New York: Oxford University Press.

Krumhansl, C. L. and Shepard, R. N. 1979. Quantification of the hierarchy of tonal functions within a diatonic context. *Journal of Experimental Psychology: Human Perception and Performance* 5(4): 579.

Kuhl, P. K., Andruski, J., Chistovich, I., *et al.* 1997. Cross-language analysis of phonetic units in language addressed to infants. *Science* 277(5326): 684–686.

Kunst, J. 1948. Around von Hornbostel's theory of the cycle of blown fifths. *Anthropos* 45(4/6): 898–900.

Kuwada, S., Batra, R., Yin, T. C., Oliver, D. L., Haberly, L. B. and Stanford, T. R. 1997. Intracellular recordings in response to monaural and binaural stimulation of neurons in the inferior colliculus of the cat. *Journal of Neuroscience* 17(19): 7565–7581.

Langner, G. 1981. Neuronal mechanisms for pitch analysis in the time domain. *Experimental Brain Research* 44: 450–454.

Langner, G. 1983. Evidence for neuronal periodicity detection in the auditory system of the guinea fowl: implications for pitch analysis in the time domain. *Experimental Brain Research* 52: 333–355.

Langner, G. 1985. Time coding and periodicity pitch. In Michelsen, A. (ed.), *Time Resolution in Auditory Systems*. Berlin: Springer: 108–121.

Langner, G. 1988. Physiological properties of units in the cochlear nucleus are adequate for a model of periodicity analysis in the auditory midbrain. In Syka, J. and Masterton, R. B. (eds), *Auditory Pathway: Structure and Function*. New York and London: Plenum Press: 207–212.

Langner, G. 1992. Periodicity coding in the auditory system. *Hearing Research* 60: 115–142.

Langner, G. 1997. Neural processing and representation of periodicity pitch. *Acta Oto-Laryngologica* 117(S532): 68–76.

Langner, G. 2004. Topographic representation of periodicity information: the 2nd neural axis of the auditory system. In Syka, J. and Merzenich, M. M. (eds), *Plasticity of the Central Auditory System and Processing of Complex Acoustic Signals*. New York and London: Plenum Press: 19–33.

Langner, G. and Scheich, H. 1978. Active phase coupling in electric fish: behavioral control with microsecond precision. *Journal of Comparative Physiology* 128: 235–240.

Langner, G. and Schreiner, C. E. 1988. Periodicity coding in the inferior colliculus of the cat: I. Neuronal mechanisms. *Journal of Neurophysiology* 60: 1799–1822.

Langner, G., Bonke, D. and Scheich, H. 1981. Neuronal discrimination of natural and synthetic vowels in field L of trained mynah birds. *Experimental Brain Research* 43(1): 11–24.

Langner, G., Decker, J., Günther, M. and Hose, B. 1987a. A computer model for periodicity analysis in the auditory midbrain based on physiological properties and connectivities of units in the cochlear nucleus. *Society for Neuroscience, Abstracts* 13(1): 546.

Langner, G., Schreiner, C. E. and Merzenich, M. M. 1987b. Covariation of latency and temporal resolution in the inferior colliculus of the cat. *Hearing Research* 31: 197–202.

Langner, G., Sams, M., Heil, P. and Schulze, H. 1997. Frequency and periodicity are represented in orthogonal maps in the human auditory cortex: evidence from magnetoencephalography. *Journal of Comparative Physiology* 181: 665–676.

Langner, G., Albert, M. and Briede, T. 2002. Temporal and spatial coding of periodicity information in the inferior colliculus of awake chinchilla (*Chinchilla laniger*). *Hearing Research* 168: 110–130.

Langner, G., Simonis, C., Braun, S. and Ochse, M. 2003. Evidence for a pitch helix in the ventral nucleus of the lateral lemniscus in the gerbil. *Association for Research in Otolaryngology, Abstracts* 26: 173.

Langner, G., Galuske, R. and Zielke, B. 2006. Three-dimensional reconstruction of the human lateral lemniscus in the auditory midbrain reveals neuronal laminae organized as a double-helix. *Forum of Neuroscience* 3: A180.9.

Langner, G., Dinse, H. R. and Godde, B. 2009. A map of periodicity orthogonal to frequency representation in the cat auditory cortex. *Frontiers in Integrative Neuroscience*, 3, doi: 10.3389/neuro.07.027.2009.

Large, E. W. and Crawford, J. D. 2002. Auditory temporal computation: interval selectivity based on post-inhibitory rebound. *Journal of Computational Neuroscience* 13(2): 125–142.

LeBeau, F. E. N., Malmierca, M. S. and Rees, A. 2001. Iontophoresis in vivo demonstrates a key role for GABA(A) and glycinergic inhibition in shaping frequency response areas in the inferior colliculus of guinea pig. *Journal of Neuroscience* 21: 7303–7312.

LeDoux, J. E. 1992. Brain mechanisms of emotion and emotional learning. *Current Opinion in Neurobiology* 2(2): 191–197.

Lesser, H. D., Frisina, R. D. and O'Neill. W. E. 1986. Responses to amplitude-modulated sounds in the inferior colliculus of the mustached bat. *Society for Neuroscience, Abstracts* 1: 1270.

Lettvin, J. Y., Maturana, H. R., McCulloch, W. S. and Pitts, W. H. 1959. What the frog's eye tells the frog's brain. *Proceedings of the IRE* 47(11): 1940–1951.

Levitin, D. J. and Rogers, S. E. 2005. Absolute pitch: perception, coding, and controversies. *Trends in Cognitive Sciences* 9(1): 26–33.

Liberman, M. C. 1978. Auditory-nerve response from cats raised in a low-noise chamber. *Journal of the Acoustical Society of America* 63: 442–445.

Licklider, J. C. R. 1941. An electrical study of frequency localization in the auditory cortex of the cat. *Psychology Bulletin* 38: 727.

Licklider, J. C. R. 1951. A duplex theory of pitch perception. *Experientia* 7: 128–134.

Liégeois-Chauvel, C., Peretz, I., Babaï, M., Laguitton, V. and Chauvel, P. 1998. Contribution of different cortical areas in the temporal lobes to music processing. *Brain* 121: 1853–1867.

Llinás, R. and Mühlethaler, M. 1988. An electrophysiological study of the in vitro, perfused brain stem-cerebellum of adult guinea-pig. *Journal of Physiology* 404: 215–240.

Loewenstein, Y., Mahon, S., Chadderton, P., *et al.* 2005. Bistability of cerebellar Purkinje cells modulated by sensory stimulation. *Nature Neuroscience* 8: 202–211.

Lorente de Nó, R. 1981. *The Primary Acoustic Nuclei*. New York: Raven.

Maier, V. 1982. Acoustic communication in the guinea fowl (*Numida meleagris*): structure and use of vocalizations, and the principles of message coding. *Zeitschrift für Tierphysiologie* 59: 29–83.

Malmierca, M. S., Leergaard, T., Bajo, V., *et al.* 1998. Anatomic evidence of a three-dimensional mosaic pattern of tonotopic organization in the ventral complex of the lateral lemniscus in cat. *Journal of Neuroscience* 18: 10603–10618.

Malmierca, M. S., Izquierdo, M. A., Cristaudo, S., *et al.* 2008. A discontinuous tonotopic organization in the inferior colliculus of the rat. *Journal of Neuroscience* 28(18): 4767–4776.

Malsburg, C. V. D. 1999. The what and why of binding: the modeler's perspective. *Neuron* 24(1): 95–104.

Malsburg, C. V. D. and Schneider, W. 1986. A neural cocktail-party processor. *Biological Cybernetics* 54: 29–40.

Mann, T. 1997. *Doctor Faustus: The Life of the German Composer Adrian Leverknotopic*. Translation by Woods, John E. New York: Alfred A. Knopf.

Margoliash, D. 2005. Song learning and sleep. *Nature Neuroscience* 8: 546–548.

Matell, M. S. and Meck, W. H. 2004. Cortico-striatal circuits and interval timing: coincidence-detection of oscillatory processes. *Cognitive Brain Research* 21: 139–170.

Maudsley, H. 1884. *Body and Will*. New York: D. Appleton and Company.

McDermott, J. and Hauser, M. 2005. The origins of music: innateness, uniqueness, and evolution. *Music Perception* 23: 29–59.

McKinney, M. F, Tramo, M. J. and Delgutte, B. 2001. Neural correlates of the dissonance of musical intervals in the inferior colliculus. In Breebaart, D. J., Houtsma, A. J. M., Kohlrausch, A., Prijs, V. F. and Schoonhoven, R. (eds), *Physiological and Psychophysical Bases of Auditory Function*. Maastricht: Shaker: 83–89.

Meddis, R. and Hewitt, M. 1991. Virtual pitch and phase sensitivity of a computer model of the auditory periphery: I. Pitch identification. *Journal of the Acoustical Society of America* 89: 2866–2882.

Meddis, R. and O'Mard, L. 1997. A unitary model of pitch perception. *Journal of the Acoustical Society of America* 102: 1811–1820.

Merchan, M. A. and Berbel, P. 1996. Anatomy of the ventral nucleus of the lateral lemniscus in rats: a nucleus with a concentric laminar organization. *Journal of Comparative Neurology* 372(2): 245–263.

Merzenich, M. M. and Reid, M. D. 1974. Representation of the cochlea within the inferior colliculus of the cat. *Brain Research* 77(3): 397–415.

Merzenich, M. M., Knight, P. L. and Roth, G. L. 1976. Representation of the cochlea within primary auditory cortex in the cat. *Journal of Neurophysiology* 38: 231–249.

Metzner, W. and Radtke-Schuller, S. 1987. The nuclei of the lateral lemniscus in the rufous horseshoe bat, *Rhinolophus rouxi*: a neurophysiological approach. *Journal of Comparative Physiology A* 160: 395–411.

Meuer, K., Wallhäusser-Franke, E. and Langner, G. 2003. Projection from inferior colliculus to the lateral lemniscus studied in a slice preparation with anterograde tracers. In Elsner, E. and Zimmermann, H. (eds), *The Neurosciences from Basic Research to Therapy*. Stuttgart: Thieme: 435–436.

Miller, M. I. and Sachs, M. B. 1984. Representation of voice pitch in discharge patterns of auditory-nerve fibers. *Hearing Research* 14(3): 257–279.

Mink, J. W. 2003. The basal ganglia and involuntary movements: impaired inhibition of competing motor patterns. *Archives of Neurology* 60: 1365–1368.

Misawa, H. and Suga, N. 2001. Multiple combination-sensitive neurons in the auditory cortex of the mustached bat. *Hearing Research* 151: 15–29.

Mogdans, J. and Knudsen, E. I. 1993. Early monaural occlusion alters the neural map of interaural level differences in the inferior colliculus of the barn owl. *Brain Research* 619: 29–38.

Møller, A. R. 1970. Two different types of frequency selective neurons in the cochlear nucleus of the rat. In Plomp, R and Smoorenburg, G. F. (eds), *Frequency Analysis and Periodicity Detection in Hearing*. Leiden: Sijthoff: 168–174.

Møller, A. R. 1971. Unit responses in the rat cochlear nucleus to tones of rapidly varing frequency and amplitude. *Acta Physiologica Scandinavica* 81: 540–556.

Møller, A. R. 1972. Coding of sounds in lower levels of the auditory system. *Quarterly Reviews of Biophysics* 5: 59–155.

Møller, A. R. 1974a. Responses of units in cochlear nucleus to sinusoidally amplitude-modulated tones. *Experimental Neurology* 45: 104–117.

Møller, A. R. 1974b. Coding of sounds with rapidly varying spectrum in the cochlear nucleus. *Journal of the Acoustical Society of America* 55: 631–640.

Møller, A. R. 1976. Dynamic properties of the responses of single neurons in the cochlear nucleus of the rat. *Journal of Physiology* 259: 63–82.

Møller, A. R. and Rees, A. 1986. Dynamic properties of the responses of single neurons in the inferior colliculus of the rat. *Hearing Research* 24: 203–215.

Montgomery, S. M. and Buzsaki, G. 2007. Gamma oscillations dynamically couple hippocampal CA3 and CA1 regions during memory task performance. *Proceedings of the National Academy of Sciences* 104: 14495–14500.

Moore, B. C. J. 1982. *An Introduction to the Psychology of Hearing*. London: Academic Press.

Moore, B. C. J., Glasberg, B. R., Flanagan, H. J. and Adams, J. 2006. Frequency discrimination of complex tones: assessing the role of component resolvability and temporal fine structure. *Journal of the Acoustical Society of America* 119(1): 480–490.

Moore, T. J. and Cashin, J. L. 1974. Response patterns of cochlear nucleus neurons to excerpts from sustained vowels. *Journal of the Acoustical Society of America* 56: 1565–1576.

Moore, T. J. and Cashin, J. L., Jr 1976. Response of cochlear-nucleus neurons to synthetic speech. *Journal of the Acoustical Society of America* 59: 1443–1449.

Moore, T. J. and Osen, K. K. 1979. The human cochlear nuclei. In Creutzfeldt, O, Scheich, H. and Schreiner, C. (eds), *Hearing Mechanisms and Speech*. Berlin: Springer: 36–44.

Morest, D. K., Kiang, N., Kane, E., Guinan, J. and Godfrey, D. 1973. Stimulus coding at caudal levels of the cat's auditory nervous system. II. Patterns of synaptic organization. In Møller, A. R. (ed.), *Basic Mechanisms in Hearing*. New York: Academic Press.

Munk, M. H., Roelfsema, P. R., König, P., Engel, A. K. and Singer, W. 1996. Role of reticular activation in the modulation of intracortical synchronization. *Science* 272(5259): 271–274.

Münzel, S., Seeberger, F. and Hein, W. 2002. The Geißenklösterle flute: discovery, experiments, reconstruction. *Studien zur Musikarchäologie* III: 107–118.

Murray, C. D. and Dermott, S. F. 1999. *Solar System Dynamics*. Cambridge: Cambridge University Press.

Musil, R. 1982. *Die Schwärmer*. Reinbek: Rowohlt.

Nelson, P. G. and Erulkar, S. D. 1963. Synaptic mechanisms of excitation and inhibition in the central auditory pathway. *Journal of Neurophysiology* 26: 908–923.

Nunez, P. L. and Shrinivasan, R. 2006. *Electric Fields of the Brain: The Neurophysics of EEG*. New York: Oxford University Press.

Ochse, M. 1999. *Intrazelluläre Ableitungen am Gehirnschnittpräparat: Untersuchungen im dorsalen Nucleus cochlearis des Gerbils* (Meriones unguiculatus). Darmstadt: TU-Darmstadt.

Ochse, M. 2005. Neuronale Kodierung von Tonhöhen und harmonischen Relationen im auditorischen Mittelhirn der Rennmaus (*Meriones unguiculatus*). PhD diss., Darmstadt: TU-Darmstadt, (http://tuprints.ulb.tu-darmstadt.de/id/eprint/524).

Ochse, M. and Langner, G. 2002. Periodizitätskodierung durch Autokorrelation und synchrone Inhibition im auditorischen Mittelhirn. *DAGA* 2: 456.

Ochse, M. and Langner, G. 2003. Modulation tuning in the auditory midbrain of gerbils: band passes are formed by inhibition. In Elsner, E. and Zimmermann, H. (eds), *The Neurosciences from Basic Research to Therapy*. Stuttgart: Thieme: 434–435.

Oertel, D. and Young, E. D. 2004. What's a cerebellar circuit doing in the auditory system? *Trends in Neurosciences* 27(2): 104–110.

Oertel, D., Wu, S. H. and Hirsch, J. A. 1988. Electrical characteristics of cells and neuronal circuitry in the cochlear nuclei studied with intracellular recording from brain slices. In Edelman, G. M., Gall, W. E. and Cowan, W. M. (eds), *Auditory Function: Neurobiological Bases of Hearing*. New York: Wiley: 313–336.

Oertel, D., Bal, R., Gardner, S., *et al.* 2000. Detection of synchrony in the activity of auditory nerve fibers by octopus cells of the mammalian cochlear nucleus. *Proceedings of the National Academy of Sciences* 97: 11773–11779.

Oertel, D., Wright, S., Cao, X. J., Ferragamo, M. and Bal, R. 2011. The multiple functions of T-stellate/multipolar/chopper cells in the ventral cochlear nucleus. *Hearing Research* 276(1): 61–69.

Oliver, D. L. 2005. Neuronal organization in the inferior colliculus. In Winer, J. A. and Schreiner, C. E. (eds), *The Inferior Colliculus*. New York: Springer: 69–114.

Oliver, D. L. and Morest, D. K. 1984. The central nucleus of the inferior colliculus in the cat. *Journal of Comparative Neurology* 222: 237–264.

Opelt, F. W. 1852. *Allgemeine Theorie der Musik auf den Rhythmus der Klangwellenpulse gegründet und durch neue Versinnlichnungsmittel erläutert*. Leipzig: Barth.

Osen, K. K. 1969. Cytoarchitecture of the cochlear nuclei in the cat. *Journal of Comparative Neurology* 136: 453–484.

Osen, K. K. 1988. Anatomy of the mammalian cochlear nuclei: a review. In Syka, J. and. Masterton, R. B. (eds), *Auditory Pathway, Structure and Function*. New York: Plenum Press: 65–75.

Palmer, A. R. 1982. Encoding of rapid amplitude fluctuations by cochlear nerve fibres in the guinea pig. *European Archives of Oto-Rhino-Laryngology* 236: 197–202.

Pantev, C., Hoke, M., Lütkenhöner, B. and Lehnertz, K. 1989. Tonotopic organization of the auditory-cortex: pitch versus frequency representation. *Science* 246: 486–488.

Parham, K. and Kim, D. O. 1995. Spontaneous and sound-evoked discharge characteristics of complex-spiking neurons in the dorsal cochlear nucleus of the unanesthetized decerebrated cat. *Journal of Neurophysiology* 73: 550–561.

Patterson, R. D. and Moore, B. C. J. 1986. Auditory filters and excitation patterns as representations of frequency resolution. In Moore, B. C. J. (ed.), *Frequency Selectivity in Hearing*. London: Academic Press: 123–177.

Pesaran, B., Pezaris, J., Sahani, M., Mitra, P. and Andersen, R. 2002. Temporal structure in neuronal activity during working memory in macaque parietal cortex. *Nature Neuroscience* 5(8): 805–811.

Peterson, G. E. and Barney, H. L. 1952. Control methods used in a study of the vowels. *Journal of the Acoustical Society of America* 24: 175–184.

Pfeiffer, R. R. 1966. Classification of response patterns of spike discharges for units in the cochlear nucleus: tone-burst stimulation. *Experimental Brain Research* 1: 220–235.

Pickles, J. O. 1988. *An Introduction to the Physiology of Hearing* (Vol. 2). London: Academic Press.

Pike, F. G., Goddard, R. S. and Suckling, J. M. 2000. Distinct frequency preferences of different types of rat hippocampal neurones in response to oscillatory input currents. *Journal of Physiology* 529(1): 205–213.

Pinker, S. 1999. How the mind works. *Annals of the New York Academy of Sciences* 882(1): 119–127.

Plack, C. J. and Oxenham, A. J. 2005. The psychophysics of pitch. In *Pitch*. New York: Springer: 7–55.

Plomp, R. and Steeneken, H. J. M. 1971. Pitch versus timbre. In *Seventh International Congress on Acoustics*, Budapest: 378–380.

Rameau, J. 1950. Ph., Traité de l'harmonie (1722). In Strunk, O. (ed.), *Source Readings in Music and History*. New York: Norton (1998).

Rauschecker, J. P. and Scott, S. K. 2009. Maps and streams in the auditory cortex: nonhuman primates illuminate human speech processing. *Nature Neuroscience* 12(6): 718–724.

Rauschecker, J. P. and Tian, B. 2000. Mechanisms and streams for processing of 'what' and 'where' in auditory cortex. *Proceedings of the National Academy of Sciences* 97: 11800–11806.

Reale, R. A. and Geisler, C. D. 1980. Auditory-nerve fiber encoding of two-tone approximations to steady-state vowels. *Journal of the Acoustical Society of America* 67(3): 891–902.

Reale, R. A. and Imig, T. J. 1980. Tonotopic organization in auditory cortex of the cat. *Journal of Comparative Neurology* 192(2): 265–291.

Rees, A. and Langner, G. 2005. Temporal coding in the auditory midbrain. In Winer, J. A. and Schreiner, C. E. (eds), *The Inferior Colliculus*. New York: Springer: 346–376.

Rees, A. and Møller, A. R. 1983. Responses of neurons in the inferior colliculus of the rat to AM and FM tones. *Hearing Research* 10(3): 301–330.

Rees, A. and Møller, A. R. 1987. Stimulus properties influencing the responses of inferior colliculus neurons to amplitude-modulated sounds. *Hearing Research* 27: 129–143.

Rees, A. and Palmer, A. R. 1989. Neuronal responses to amplitude-modulated and pure-tone stimuli in the guinea pig inferior colliculus, and their modification by broad-band noise. *Journal of the Acoustical Society of America* 85: 1978–1994.

Reimer, K. 1987. Coding of sinusoidally amplitude modulated acoustic stimuli in the inferior colliculus of the rufous horseshoe bat, *Rhinolophus rouxi. Journal of Comparative Physiology* A161: 305–313.

Reinhold, N., Kuehnel, S., Brand, M. and Markowitsch, H. J. 2006. Functional neuroimaging in memory and memory disturbances. *Current Medical Imaging Reviews* 2(1): 35–57.

Rhode, W. S. 1994. Temporal coding of 200% amplitude modulated signals in the ventral cochlear nucleus of cat. *Hearing Research* 77: 43–68.

Rhode, W. S. 1998. Neural encoding of single-formant stimuli in the ventral cochlear nucleus of the chinchilla. *Hearing Research* 117: 39–56.

Rhode, W. S. 1999. Vertical cell responses to sound in cat dorsal cochlear nucleus. *Journal of Neurophysiology* 82: 1019–1032.

Rhode, W. S. and Greenberg, S. 1994. Encoding of amplitude modulation in the cochlear nucleus of the cat. *Journal of Neurophysiology* 71: 1797–1825.

Rhode, W. S. and Smith, P. H. 1986. Encoding timing and intensity in the ventral cochlear nucleus of the cat. *Journal of Neurophysiology* 56: 261–286.

Rhode, W. S., Smith, P. H. and Oertel, D. 1983a. Physiological response properties of cells labeled intracellularly with horseradish peroxidase in cat dorsal cochlear nucleus. *Journal of Comparative Neurology* 213: 426–447.

Rhode, W. S., Oertel, D. and Smith, P. H. 1983b. Physiological response properties of cells labeled intracellularly with horseradish peroxidase in cat ventral cochlear nucleus. *Journal of Comparative Neurology* 213: 448–463.

Rieger, M. 2006. *Helmholtz Musicus. Die Objektivierung der Musik im 19. Jahrhundert durch Helmholtz' Lehre von den Tonempfindungen.* Darmstadt: WBG.

Riquelme, R., Saldaña, E., Osen, K. K., Ottersen, O. P. and Merchán, M. A. 2001. Colocalization of GABA and glycine in the ventral nucleus of the lateral lemniscus in rat: an in situ hybridization and semiquantitative immunocytochemical study. *Journal of Comparative Neurology* 432(4): 409–424.

Ritsma, R. J. 1967. Frequencies dominant in the perception of pitch of complex sounds. *Journal of the Acoustical Society of America* 42: 191–198.

Ritsma, R. J. 1970. Periodicity detection. In Plomp, R. and Smoorenburg, G. F. (eds), *Frequency Analysis and Periodicity Detection in Hearing.* Leiden: Sijthoff: 250–266.

Rockel, A. J. and Jones, E. G. 1973. The neuronal organization of the inferior colliculus of the adult cat: I. The central nucleus. *Journal of Comparative Neurology* 147: 11–60.

Rolls, E. T., Critchley, H. D., Browning, A. S. and Inoue, K. 2006. Face-selective and auditory neurons in the primate orbitofrontal cortex. *Experimental Brain Research* 170(1): 74–87.

Rose, G. J. and Capranica, R. R. 1985. Sensitivity to amplitude modulated sounds in the anuran auditory nervous system. *Journal of Neurophysiology* 53: 446–465.

Rose, J. E., Hind, J. E., Anderson, D. J. and Brugge, J. F. 1971. Some effects of stimulus intensity on response of auditory nerve fibers in the squirrel monkey. *Journal of Neurophysiology* 34(4): 685–699.

Rossing, T. D. 1989. *The Science of Sound.* Reading, MA: Addison Wesley.

Rouiller, E. M. and Ryugo, D. K. 1984. Intracellular marking of physiologically characterized cells in the ventral cochlear nucleus of the cat. *Journal of Comparative Neurology* 225: 167–186.

Ruggero, M. A. and Rich, N. C. 1987. Timing of spike initiation in cochlear afferents: dependance on site of innervation. *Journal of Neurophysiology* 58: 379–403.

Rupert, A. L. R., Caspary, D. M. and Moushegian, G. 1977. Response characteristics of cochlear nucleus neurons to vowel sounds. *Annals of Otology, Rhinology, and Laryngology* 86: 37–48.

Sabatini, B. L. and Regehr, W. G. 1999. Timing of synaptic transmission. *Annual Review of Physiology* 61(1): 521–542.

Sachs, M. and Kiang, N. Y. C. 1968. Two-tone inhibition in auditory nerve fibers. *Journal of the Acoustical Society of America* 43: 1120–1128.

Sachs, M. B. and Young, E. D. 1979. Encoding of steady-state vowels in the auditory nerve: representation in terms of discharge rate. *Journal of the Acoustical Society of America* 66: 470–479.

Sachs, M. B., Blackburn, C. and Young, E. D. 1988. Rate-place and temporal-place representations of vowels in the auditory nerve and anteroventral cochlear nucleus. *Journal of Phonetics* 16: 37–53.

Scheich, H., Langner, G. and Koch, R. 1977. Coding of narrow-band and wide-band vocalizations in the auditory midbrain nucleus (MLD) of the guinea fowl (*Numida meleagris*). *Journal of Comparative Physiology* 117: 245–265.

Scheich, H., Bock, W., Bonke, D., Langner, G. and Maier, V. 1983. Acoustic communication in the guinea fowl (*Numida meleagris*). In *Advances in Vertebrate Neuroethology*. New York: Springer: 731–782.

Schildberger, K. 1984. Temporal selectivity of identified auditory neurons in the cricket brain. *Journal of Comparative Physiology* 155: 171–186.

Schneider, P., Sluming, V., Roberts, N., *et al.* 2005. Structural and functional asymmetry of lateral Heschl's gyrus reflects pitch perception preference. *Nature Neuroscience* 8(9): 1241–1247.

Schofield, B. R. and Cant, N. B. 1997. Ventral nucleus of the lateral lemniscus in guinea pigs: cytoarchitecture and inputs from the cochlear nucleus. *Journal of Comparative Neurology* 379: 363–385.

Schouten, J. F. 1938. The perception of subjective tones. *Proceedings of Koninklijke Nederlandse Akademie van Wetenschappen* 41: 1086–1093.

Schouten, J. F. 1940a. The perception of pitch. *Philips Technical Review* 5: 286–294.

Schouten, J. F. 1940b. The residue, a new component in subjective sound analysis. *Proceedings of Koninklijke Nederlandse Akademie van Wetenschappen* 43: 356–365.

Schouten, J. F. 1970. The residue revisited. In Plomp, R. and Smoorenburg, G. F. (eds), *Frequency Analysis and Periodicity Detection in Hearing*. Leiden: Sijthoff: 41–54.

Schouten, J. F., Ritsma, R. J. and Cardozo, B. L. 1962. Pitch of the residue. *Journal of the Acoustical Society of America* 34: 1418–1424.

Schreiner, C. E. and Langner, G. 1988. Coding of temporal patterns in the central auditory nervous system. In Edelmann, G. M., Gall, W. E. and Cowan, W. M. (eds), *Auditory Function*. New York: J. Wiley & Sons: 337–361.

Schreiner, C. E. and Langner, G. 1997. Laminar fine structure of frequency organization in auditory midbrain. *Nature* 388: 383–386.

Schreiner, C. E. and Mendelson, J. R. 1990. Functional topography of cat primary auditory cortex: distribution of integrated excitation. *Journal of Neurophysiology* 64: 1442–1459.

Schreiner, C. E. and Snyder, R. 1987. Modulation transfer characteristics of neurons in the dorsal cochlear nucleus of the cat. *Society for Neuroscience, Abstracts* 13: 1258.

Schreiner, C. E., Urbas, J. V. and Mehrgardt, S. 1983. Temporal resolution of amplitude modulation and complex signals in the auditory cortex of the cat. In Klinke, R. and Hartmann, R. (eds), *Hearing: Physiological Bases and Psychophysics*. Berlin: Springer: 169–175.

Schreiner, C. E., Read, H. L. and Sutter, M. L. 2000. Modular organization of frequency integration in primary auditory cortex. *Annual Review of Neuroscience* 23(1): 501–529.

Schroeder, C. E. and Lakatos, P. 2009. Low-frequency neuronal oscillations as instruments of sensory selection. *Trends in Neuroscience* 32: 9–18.

Schuller, G. 1979. Coding of small sinusoidal frequency and amplitude modulations in the inferior colliculus of the 'CF-FM' bat, *Rhinolophus ferrumequinum*. *Experimental Brain Research* 34: 117–132.

Schulze, H. and Langner, G. 1999. Representation of signal periodicity in the auditory cortex. *Zeitschrift für Audiologie* II: 7–12.

Schulze, H., Hess, A., Ohl, F. W. and Scheich, H. 2002. Superposition of horseshoe-like periodicity and linear tonotopic maps in auditory cortex of the Mongolian gerbil. *European Journal of Neuroscience* 15(6): 1077–1084.

Schwarz, D. W. F. and Tomlinson, R. W. W. 1990. Spectral response patterns of auditory-cortex neurons to harmonic complex tones in alert monkey (*Macaca-mulatta*). *Journal of Neurophysiology* 64: 282–298.

Seebeck, A. 1844. Über die Definition des Tones. *Annalen der Physik* 139: 353–368.

Semal, C. and Demany, L. 1990. The upper limit of musical pitch. *Music Perception* 8: 165–175.

Shadlen, M. N. and Movshon, J. A. 1999. Synchrony unbound: a critical evaluation of the temporal binding hypothesis. *Neuron* 24: 67–77.

Shepard, R. N. 1982. Geometrical approximations to the structure of musical pitch. *Psychological Review* 89(4): 305–333.

Shivapuja, B. G. R., Salvi, J. and Saunders, S. S. 1990. Response of auditory-nerve fibers to intensity increments in a multitone complex: neural correlates of profile analysis. *Journal of the Acoustical Society of America* 88: 2211–2221.

Shore, S. E. and Zhou, J. 2006. Somatosensory influence on the cochlear nucleus and beyond. *Hearing Research* 216: 90–99.

Sinex, D. G. and Geisler, C. D. 1983. Responses of auditory-nerve fibers to consonant-vowel syllables. *Journal of the Acoustical Society of America* 73: 602–615.

Singer, W. 1999. Neuronal synchrony: a versatile code for the definition of relations? *Neuron* 24: 49.

Singer, W. 2001. Consciousness and the binding problem. *Annals of the New York Academy of Sciences* 929(1): 123–146.

Singer, W. 2007. Binding by synchrony. *Scholarpedia* 2(12): 1657.

Singer, W. 2013. Cortical dynamics revisited. *Trends in Cognitive Sciences* 17(12): 616–626.

Smith, R. L. 1979. Adaptation, saturation, and physiological masking in single auditory-nerve fibers. *Journal of the Acoustical Society of America* 650: 1660–1780.

Spirou, G. A., Davis, K. A., Nelken, I. and Young, E. D. 1999. Spectral integration by type II interneurons in dorsal cochlear nucleus. *Journal of Neurophysiology* 82: 648–663.

Stauffer, E. K., Watt, D. G., Taylor, A., Reinking, R. M. and Stuart, D. G. 1976. Analysis of muscle receptor connections by spike-triggered averaging: 2. Spindle group II afferents. *Journal of Neurophysiology* 39(6): 1393–1402.

Stein, A. von and Sarnthein, J. 2000. Different frequencies for different scales of cortical integration: from local gamma to long range alpha/theta synchronization. *International Journal of Psychophysiology* 38(3): 301–313.

Stiebler, J. and Ehret, G. 1985. Inferior colliculus of the house mouse: I. A quantitative study tonotopic organization, frequency representation, and tone-threshold representation. *Journal of Comparative Neurology* 238: 65–76.

Stokkum, I. H. M. V. 1987. Sensitivity of neurons in the dorsal medullary nucleus of the grassfrog to spectral and temporal characteristics of sound. *Hearing Research* 29: 223–235.

Stokkum, I. H. M. V. and Gielen, C. C. A. M. 1989. A model for the peripheral auditory nervous system of the grassfrog. *Hearing Research* 41(1): 71–85.

Stryker, M. P. 1989. Is grandmother an oscillation? *Nature* 338: 297–298.

Stumpf, C. 1890. *Tonpsychologie*. Leipzig: Hirzel.

Stumpf, C. 1939. *Erkenntnislehre* (Vol. I). Leipzig: Barth.

Stumpf, C. 1940. *Erkenntnislehre* (Vol. II). Leipzig: Barth.

Suga, N. and O'Neill, W. E. 1979. Neural axis representing target range in the auditory cortex of the mustache bat. *Science* 206(4416): 351–353.

Suga, N. and Schlegel, P. 1972. Analysis of information-bearing elements in complex sounds by auditory neurons of bats. *Audiology* 11: 58–72.

Suga, N. and Schlegel, P. 1973. Coding and processing in the auditory systems of the FM-signal-producing bats. *Journal of the Acoustical Society of America* 54: 174–190.

Suga, N., Gao, E., Zhang, Y., Ma, X. and Olsen, J. F. 2000. The corticofugal system for hearing: recent progress. *Proceedings of the National Academy of Sciences* 97(22): 11807–11814.

Swindale, N. V. 2004. How different feature spaces may be represented in cortical maps. *Network: Computation in Neural Systems* 15(4): 217–242.

Tallon-Baudry, C., Bertrand, O., Peronnet, F. and Pernier, J. 1998. Induced γ-band activity during the delay of a visual short-term memory task in humans. *Journal of Neuroscience* 18(11): 4244–4254.

Terhardt, E. 1972a. Zur Tonhöhenwahrnehmung von Klängen I. Psychoakustische Grundlagen. *Acustica* 26: 174–186.

Terhardt, E. 1972b. Zur Tonhöhenwahrnehmung von Klängen II. Ein Funktionsschema. *Acustica* 26: 187–199.

Terhardt, E. 1991. Music perception and sensory information acquisition: relationships and low-level analogies. *Music Perception* 8: 217–240.

Thomas, H., Tillein, J., Heil, P. and Scheich, H. 1993. Functional organization of auditory cortex in the Mongolian gerbil (*Meriones unguiculatus*): I. Electrophysiological mapping of frequency representation and distinction of fields. *European Journal of Neuroscience* 5: 882–897.

Tiesinga, P. H., Fellous, J. M., Salinas, E., José, J. V. and Sejnowski, T. J. 2004. Inhibitory synchrony as a mechanism for attentional gain modulation. *Journal of Physiology* 98(4–6): 296–314.

Tonndorf, J. 1960. Shearing motion in scala media of cochlear models. *Journal of the Acoustical Society of America* 32(2): 238–244.

Torbett, M., Greenberg, R. and Smoluchowski, R. 1982. Orbital resonances and planetary formation sites. *Icarus* 49: 313–326.

Trainor, L. J., Tsang, C. D. and Cheung, V. H. W. 2002. Preference for sensory consonance in 2- and 4-month-old infants. *Music Perception* 20: 187–194.

Tramo, M. J., Cariani, P. A., Delgutte, B. and Braida, L. D. 2001. Neurobiological foundations for the theory of harmony in western tonal music. *Annals of the New York Academy of Sciences* 930: 92–116.

Treurniet, W. C. and Boucher, D. R. 2001. A masking level difference due to harmonicity. *Journal of the Acoustical Society of America* 109: 306–320.

Tunturi, A. R. 1944. Audiofrequency localization in the acoustic cortex of the dog. *American Journal of Physiology* 141: 397–403.

Turner, R. S. 1977. The Ohm–Seebeck dispute, Hermann von Helmholtz, and the origins of physiological acoustics. *British Journal for the History of Science* 10: 1–24.

Tyndall, J. 1893. *Sound*. London: Longmans, Green, and Co.

Ueda, K. and Ohgushi, K. 1987. Perceptual components of pitch: spatial representation using a multidimensional scaling technique. *Journal of the Acoustical Society of America* 82: 1193–1200.

Uhlhaas, P. J., Haenschel, C., Nikolić, D. and Singer, W. 2008. The role of oscillations and synchrony in cortical networks and their putative relevance for the pathophysiology of schizophrenia. *Schizophrenia Bulletin* 34(5): 927–943.

Vater, M. 1982. Single unit responses in cochlear nucleus of horseshoe bats to sinusoidal frequency and amplitude modulated signals. *Journal of Comparative Physiology* 149: 369–388.

Vater, M., Habbicht, H., Kössl, M. and Grothe, B. 1992. The functional-role of GABA and glycine in monaural and binaural processing in the inferior colliculus of horseshoe bats. *Journal of Comparative Physiology* 171: 541–553.

Vater, M., Covey, E. and Casseday, J. H. 1997. The columnar region of the ventral nucleus of the lateral lemniscus in the big brown bat (*Eptesicus fuscus*): synaptic arrangements and structural correlates of feedforward inhibitory function. *Cell and Tissue Research* 289(2): 223–233.

Voigt, H. F. and Young, E. D. 1990. Cross-correlation analysis of inhibitory interactions in dorsal cochlear nucleus. *Journal of Neurophysiology* 64: 1590–1610.

Voutsas, K. and Adamy, J. 2005. A biologically inspired spiking neural network for sound source localization. *IEEE Transactions on Neural Networks* 18: 1785–1799.

Walkowiak, W. 1984. Neuronal correlates of the recognition of pulsed sound signals in the grass frog. *Journal of Comparative Physiology* 155: 57–66.

Walton, J. P., Frisina, R. D. and O'Neill, W. E. 1998. Age-related alteration in processing of temporal sound features in the auditory midbrain of the CBA mouse. *Journal of Neuroscience* 18: 2764–2776.

Ward, W. D. 1999. Absolute pitch. In Deutsch, D. (ed.), *The Psychology of Music*. New York: Academic Press: 265–298.

Warr, W. B. 1982. Parallel ascending pathways from the cochlear nucleus: neuroanatomical evidence of functional specialization. In Neff, W. D. (ed.), *Sensory Physiology*. New York: Academic Press: 1–38.

Warren, B., Gibson, G. and Russell, I. J. 2009. Sex recognition through midflight mating duets in *Culex* mosquitoes is mediated by acoustic distortion. *Current Biology* 19(6): 485–491.

Watkins, S., Shams, L., Josephs, O. and Rees, G. 2007. Activity in human V1 follows multisensory perception. *Neuroimage* 37(2): 572–578.

Wenstrup, J. J. and Grose, C. D. 1995. Inputs to combination-sensitive neurons in the medial geniculate body of the mustached bat: the missing fundamental. *Journal of Neuroscience* 15: 4693–4711.

Wernicke, C. 1874. *Der aphasische Sypmtomenkomplex eine psychologische Studie auf anatomischer Basis*. Breslau: Hohn and Weigert.

Wever, E. G. 1949. *Theory of Hearing*. New York: Wiley.

Whittington, M. A. and Traub, R. D. 2003. Interneuron diversity series: inhibitory interneurons and network oscillations in vitro. *Trends in Neuroscience* 26: 676–682.

Wickesberg, R. E. and Oertel, D. 1990. Delayed frequency-specific inhibition in the cochlear nuclei of mice: a mechanism for monaural echo suppression. *Journal of Neuroscience* 10: 1762–1768.

Wightman, F. L. 1973. The pattern-transformation model of pitch. *Journal of the Acoustical Society of America* 54: 407–416.

Willard, F. H. and Martin, G. F. 1983. The auditory brainstem nuclei and some of their projections to the inferior colliculus in the North American opossum. *Neuroscience* 10(4): 1203–1232.

Willott, J. F. and Bross, L. S. 1990. Morphology of the octopus cell area of the cochlear nucleus in young and aging C57BL/6J and CBA/J mice. *Journal of Comparative Neurology* 300: 61–81.

Winter, I. M., Robertson, D. and Yates, G. K. 1990. Diversity of characteristic frequency rate-intensity functions in guinea pig auditory nerve fibres. *Hearing Research* 45: 191–202.

Winter, P. and Funkenstein, H. H. 1973. The effect of species-specific vocalizations on the discharge of auditory cortical cells in the awake squirrel monkey (*Saimiri sciureus*). *Experimental Brain Research* 18: 489–504.

Woolsey, C. G. and Walzl, E. M. 1942. Topical projection of nerve fibers from local regions of the cochlea to the cerebral cortex of the cat. *Bulletin of the Johns Hopkins Hospital* 71: 315–344.

Wu, S. H. 1999. Physiological properties of neurons in the ventral nucleus of the lateral lemniscus of the rat: intrinsic membrane properties and synaptic responses. *Journal of Neurophysiology* 81(6): 2862–2874.

Xu, L. and Pfingst, B. E. 2008. Spectral and temporal cues for speech recognition: implications for auditory prostheses. *Hearing Research* 242(1–2): 132–140.

Yost, W. A. and Sheft, S. 1994. Modulation detection interference: across-frequency processing and auditory grouping. *Hearing Research* 79: 48–58.

Young, E. D. and Brownell, W. E. 1976. Responses to tones and noise of single cells in dorsal cochlear nucleus of unanesthetized cats. *Journal of Neurophysiology* 39: 282–300.

Young, E. D. and Sachs, M. B. 1979. Representation of steady state vowels in the temporal aspects of the discharge patterns of populations of auditory nerve fibers. *Journal of the Acoustical Society of America* 66: 1381–1403.

Young, E. D., Robert, J. M. and Shofner, W. P. 1988. Regularity and latency of units in ventral cochlear nucleus: implications for unit classification and generation of response properties. *Journal of Neurophysiology* 60: 1–29.

Zatorre, R. 2003. Music and the brain. *Annals of the New York Academy of Sciences* 999: 4–14.

Zatorre, R. J. and Samson, S. 1991. Role of the right temporal neocortex in retention of pitch in auditory short-term memory. *Brain* 114(6): 2403–2417.

Zatorre, R. J., Chen, J. L. and Penhune, V. B. 2007. When the brain plays music: auditory–motor interactions in music perception and production. *Nature Reviews Neuroscience* 8(7): 547–558.

Zhang, D. X., Li, L., Kelly, J. B. and Wu, S. H. 1998. GABAergic projections from the lateral lemniscus to the inferior colliculus of the rat. *Hearing Research* 117(1): 1–12.

Zhang, H. and Kelly, J. B. 2006. Responses of neurons in the rat's ventral nucleus of the lateral lemniscus to amplitude-modulated tones. *Journal of Neurophysiology* 96(6): 2905–2914.

Zhang, S. and Oertel, D. 1993. Giant cells of the dorsal cochlear nucleus of mice: intracellular recordings in slices. *Journal of Neurophysiology* 69(5): 1398–1408.

Zhao, H. B. and Liang, Z. A. 1995. Processing of modulation frequency in the dorsal cochlear nucleus of the guinea pig: amplitude modulated tones. *Hearing Research* 82(2): 244–256.

Zhao, M. and Wu, S. H. 2001. Morphology and physiology of neurons in the ventral nucleus of the lateral lemniscus in rat brain slices. *Journal of Comparative Neurology* 433(2): 255–271.

Zhou, N., Huang, J., Chen, X. and Xu, L. 2013. Relationship between tone perception and production in prelingually deafened children with cochlear implants. *Otology & Neurotology* 34: 499–506.

Zschau, C. 2008. Einfluß von Lautstärke und Modulationstiefe auf die Periodizitätsverarbeitung im Colliculus inferior der Mongolischen Wüstenrennmaus (*Meriones unguiculatus*). Thesis, Darmstadt: TU-Darmstadt.

Zwicker, E. and Feldtkeller, R. 1967. *Das Ohr als Nachrichtenempfänger*. Stuttgart: S. Hirzel Verlag.

Zwicker, E., Flottorp, G. and Stevens, S. 1957. Critical band width in loudness summation. *Journal of the Acoustical Society of America* 29: 548–557.

Index